Burdened to Tell

Burdened *to* Tell

Sharon E. Allen

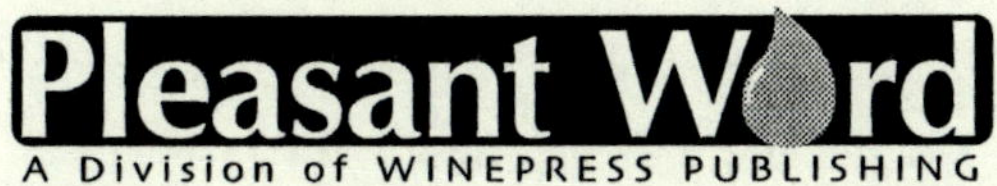

Contents

ACKNOWLEDGEMENTS

Any undertaking of this nature requires help and understanding from others. To **Patricia A. Campbell** I am deeply indebted for her painstaking review and corrections of the original manuscript. To **Patricia Kennedy** I am grateful for reading the manuscript and providing her opinions. Also, I must thank **Sheila Bartley** for her expertise with my computer. To **Anita**, I just say thank you!

Chapter 1

IT'S CANCER!

On August 28, 2001, an ear, nose, and throat (ENT) surgeon removed a tumor located high in my ethmoid sinuses, the area behind the eyes at the base of the frontal lobe of the brain. Only the usual anxiety that surrounds any surgery was there, since ninety percent of growths in this area are benign. Unfortunately, there are ten percent that have to make up the remainder.

When I received information that I fell in the latter group, there was the usual fear and trauma that goes with the word cancer. The physician was extremely attentive. He called me personally to let me know what was going on. Additionally, he told me that the hospital where the surgery had taken place identified the tumor as "spindle cell," but they were unable to further specify the type. Therefore, the frozen sections of the tumor were sent to Mayo Clinic in Rochester, Minnesota, for confirmation. It was indeed a spindle cell tumor, further identified as a synovial sarcoma. This diagnosis was not good. This is an extremely rare form of cancer in the head region, particularly in the sinuses. It appeared a death knell had sounded.

Great interest arose as a result of the unusual location of this tumor. The surgeon referred me to a well-known medical school in a nearby city since they were close and had a large staff to investigate the situation. A cancer center about 250 miles away also expressed interest in the investigation and wanted some of its staff involved as well because of the rarity of the tumor and its location. Tests, tests, and more tests followed. MRI machines became more familiar than my home. I saw more doctors and technicians over the period of a few days' time than I had seen in many years. I had never heard of a "tumor board." However, I learned that this was a group of physicians (in my case, neurosurgeons, ENT physicians, oncologists, etc.) who set aside a half day to discuss all test results and determine their best assessment for treatment.

One of the medical school surgeons had told me about proton beam radiation. He suggested the possibility that it might be a recommended treatment for me. He would know more after meeting with others on the tumor board when all tests were completed. Two locations in the U.S. provided this radiation treatment. One was located in the northeastern U.S. and the other in southern California. Having cancer was a bummer, but southern California in the winter was not the worst thing to think about. As bad as cancer is, perhaps mixing the pleasure of a warm winter with treatment could provide some comfort.

Only a few days after the cancer diagnosis, I felt comfortable with my prayer life, relative to the matter and told family and friends that the Lord would let me know what course I was to take. So many tests! I was still recuperating from surgery. Then, interestingly, the school counselor who had worked with me more than twenty years earlier when I had once been a school principal, called me the evening before the tumor board was to meet. We had worked together many years before, and it was quite a coincidence that she called since our lives had moved in far different directions. In fact, I was retired and living in a city seventy miles away. During the course of our conversation, she informed me that only a year earlier her daughter-in-law had a malignant tumor removed that was located somewhere near her throat area. She had received radiation therapy after removal of the tumor. She was young, in her twenties. The counselor told me that radiation therapy in and around the face can have devastating results. Her daughter-in-law carried a bottle of water around at all times in order to get enough moisture to speak since her salivary glands no longer produced saliva. She had a feeding tube in order to get nourishment. Through it all, the daughter-in-law was grateful that she was alive to rear her children.

I had felt so positive that I would know what I should do when the doctor called the following morning, but worry crept in when I considered the information I received about radiation and that a definite answer had not come from the Lord! On the morning that the tumor board was to meet, I asked the Lord why there had not been an answer. His timing is always perfect—where was He? I never considered the phone call the night before being anything other than coincidence.

The phone rang: it was the physician with information from the "think tank." When I heard the recommendation, the answer from the Lord was there. It was as if He said "No way!" It was on a Thursday, and the doctor asked me to wait until after the weekend and to think it over. He would call again on Monday. I attempted to assure him that my decision was in response to prayer and my belief that the Lord had given me this answer when I heard his recommendation.

This physician informed me that my cancer was a type that moves very rapidly once disturbed. Its nature is to crumble into many pieces when touched. The surgeon who had removed it had provided me with information that it had indeed crumbled during removal. He informed me that he had scraped it off the bone that lies beneath the frontal lobe of my brain. Additionally, it had grown against my spinal cord, Eustachian tube, and right optic nerve. He had also been most aggressive with my olfactory organs as he performed the surgery. To have completely removed all pieces of the tumor would have been virtually impossible.

I was informed by the medical school doctor that the physicians who comprised the tumor board had determined the best course of treatment to be further surgery first, followed by radiation. Surgery was to consist of removing my "skull cap," then lifting the frontal lobe of my brain out while removing the bone that lies beneath it, then graft new bone in its place. After this was completed, the frontal lobe would be replaced and my skull sewn back on. This surgery would then be followed by several radiation treatments. The prognosis would be a forty percent chance of total cure and a sixty percent chance of buying five to seven years in remission.

As I listened, I was in shock, I think. From the moment I recovered originally after being told that the tumor was malignant, I had envisioned a recommendation of chemotherapy, radiation, or both. Additionally, I had prayed without ceasing about what I should do were I given options. Surgery of the magnitude he proposed could not have entered my mind. Actually, I had not thought about further surgery at all!

On Monday, the call came and my response was the same. The doctor seemed shocked that I refused treatment. He suggested that since my concern was for the surgery, perhaps chemotherapy followed by radiation would be more acceptable to me. That would be far better than accepting a death sentence. (He did not use these latter words, but they were obvious.) His final words were to let me know that he and all those involved were certainly interested in my well-being. Further, if at any time I had any need, to feel free to call. I almost wanted to be on the other end of the phone to console this wonderful person. Although I was confident the Lord was in charge of my refusal for treatment, it was difficult to close the door to these wonderful and caring health professionals. In this day when we are so often reminded that doctors are overburdened with paperwork and other pressures from insurance companies that their patients receive inferior attention, the opposite was represented in this situation. Indeed it is a medical school, indeed they conduct research and write papers, but in and through it all, they were kind, loving and empathetic.

The original ENT who had operated on me continued with follow-up care. He seemed to understand my position. It was appointed that I return for a six-month checkup for him to perform an endoscopy (an instrument was inserted through my nose into my ethmoid sinuses located behind and between my eyes) to see if there was anything growing in the area where the tumor had been removed. As I sat while this procedure was taking place, it seemed that the physician was taking forever to make a comment as he looked around inside my head. At long last he said, "Humph!" I waited for more. Nothing came. I could not stand it. I asked, "Was that a good humph, or a bad humph?" After another long pause, he responded "It's clean as a whistle." This is a busy physician, but he was very kind and talked with me for several minutes without the appearance that he needed to move on. Before I left, he said, "It will be interesting if nothing else shows up and I wanted to take your body apart." He did inform me that the only definitive way to know whether anything was there was to see an MRI of my head. He said the greatest worries were for the bone beneath the brain (where he had scraped tumor pieces) and the optic nerve of my right eye. I requested that we wait for six months to complete the MRI. He seemed hesitant but complied (The hesitance may have been a response of surprise for not visibly finding anything growing, since most accounts point out that synovial sarcoma "hosts" die within seven or eight months of removal of an untreated tumor.). Being a good physician, he wanted to be sure nothing was there.

One of the concerns had been recurrence in my right optic nerve. The day after the appointment with the surgeon, I had an appointment with my ophthalmologist. When I went for the ophthalmologist visit, I told her about the tumor removal six months before. She was most interested and took pains to look at my right optic nerve. After what again seemed a very long time, she said, "Your optic nerve is pink, pulsating, and very healthy looking." Wow, what news!

Six months down, everything was positive. All information on the Internet relative to this cancer gave a dismal prognosis. In every case, death came in seven or eight months time, treated or untreated. It would be untrue to say there had been no anxiety during the past six months, but actually, it had been the best six months of my life. When I would tell someone it was the best six months of my life, he would respond with either disbelief or think me a saint. As you will learn later, sainthood was not anywhere in the equation. All through my life, the Lord had played a vital though sometimes distant role, but my relationship grew so much closer during this six months that His nearness and position of Lord were definite.

During the next six months there were times I thought about the MRI to come, but for the most part, I believed God had healed me. After the six months had passed, and it was time for the MRI, I felt wonderful physically, and emotionally, there was only a little anxiety. There was a two-week wait between the actual test and my review with the doctor. However, a few days after the MRI, there was a message on the recorder when I returned home one day. It said, "This is Cindy from the doctor's office. Your MRI is normal. The doctor wants to see you anyway." Wow, a normal MRI! Now what?

Chapter 2

ORIGINAL SYMPTOMS

The question always comes, "How did you know there was a problem?" We always want to know what another's symptoms were so we may avoid those pitfalls. In my case, the symptoms were vague and non-dramatic. It was perhaps in 1995 or 1996 that I went to see an internist about a strange feeling in my right ear. There was no problem with hearing, no true discomfort, no pain. An allergy-related problem was suspected and the drug Sudafed probably would take care of it. I took Sudafed for a week or so and experienced no change.

Several months later, I went to another internist with the same complaint and an additional concern that had developed since the visit with the last doctor. This time, I had a large swelling in my right salivary gland. I was referred to an ENT who was young and very attentive. There was an obvious problem with the salivary gland, which he told me was not uncommon. If it continued to be a bother, surgery could correct the problem. While I was there, I mentioned the vague feeling I had in my right ear and the earlier visit to a doctor in another city. I asked if there might be a connection with using a cell phone. (My job had afforded many hours of cell phone use and comments were being made on television and in other media concerning possible use of cell phones and brain tumors.) This question was probably too far out for any serious thought but the news media had gotten my attention. The physician expressed no concern. I was to monitor my salivary gland swelling, and if it became bothersome, he could perform a simple surgery and eliminate the problem. In addition, the next time the gland became really swollen, I was to call immediately to get a CT scan.

Probably about five years later, in January of 2001, I went to see a well-respected ENT I had seen for a routine problem in the early 1990's. I had had no further problems with my salivary gland; however, the strange feeling in my right ear remained after all those years. Cell phone connections with brain tumors were being discussed again, and I wanted an answer. The physician examined me for less than two minutes, gave me a prescription for the drug Flonase and sent me on my way. By the way, I asked him about the possibility of a tumor, and he suggested that the prescription spray he was prescribing would shrink anything that might be causing my problem.

In February of 2001, I went to see my ophthalmologist and explained that I was feeling a strange sensation in my right eye. I knew this doctor was a good one, but I didn't risk the cell phone comments or the many-year chase of the vague feeling. She thoroughly examined my eye and told me my vitreous humor, the liquid part of the eye that flecks, causing black spots as we age, was interfering with my vision. When I left her office, I felt confident that there was not a problem with my eye. She was attentive and thorough. Had I mentioned my other concerns, I am confident she would have investigated with a CT or MRI and found the problem, but I did not. Since my right optic nerve was not damaged by the tumor's presence, she was unable to detect the presence of a tumor.

Two or three months later, during a routine pap test with my gynecologist, I told him about all the visits I had made about my ear and that I guessed it must not be anything to worry about. He asked if I ever had bad headaches. I told him that on occasion I had headaches, not usually that severe. Many years before, I had been told I had migraine "auras," but the headaches never materialized. The gynecologist suggested I see a neurologist. The gynecologist knew someone he wanted me to see.

Well, I guess the rest is history. I saw the neurologist, and he sent me to have several things checked. He sent me to an orthopedic surgeon because the MRI he ordered showed spondylosis, a fancy word for deteriorating bone, of the lower spine and neck. He sent me to a cardiologist because he needed information in order to rule out any cardiovascular problems that would preclude his prescribing a migraine medication. He sent me to an ENT because the MRI of my head showed a large mass in "no man's land" of the ethmoid sinuses, leaning toward the right.

One thing I have surely learned: it is most important to have an internist or general practitioner who knows you, your body, and your personality. Without the gynecologist who knew me and believed I needed to see a neurologist to investigate my symptoms, the tumor might have invaded my bone and brain tissue. However, it might be said that the Lord's timing is always perfect. Therefore, I will have to wait until I see Him to know for sure! At any rate, I am in the process at this writing of developing a rapport with an internist in the town where I live.

THE TROUBLED BEGINNING

You know about my cancer and how it was found. What about the person who had it? I was born in early June of 1944, to middle-class parents in Texas. My parents were devout Southern Baptists during a time marked by strict behavior at home, at church, and at school. My parents loved their children, wanted the best for them, and were willing to sacrifice whatever it took for them to be fed, clothed, and educated. What adults said ruled; children were to be seen and not heard. Today, I see my mother as a sweet, smiling angel. Growing up, I saw a nagging, unrelenting person whom everyone else thought was wonderful. I recognized her love, but what she called her standards kept me away. My dad and I were very close, but I was careful to insure he did not become angry with me. As I look back now, I realize that in that time, Southern Baptists were very law oriented, even more so than today. Add to that a family requirement for perfection. There was no room for even a hint of laziness and no room for doing less than your very best. Failure of any kind was to be avoided at all costs; if it happened, it needed to be kept in the family and never repeated. Although I realize pride to be one of the great downfalls of man, it seemed to be a *good* thing in our household.

Before starting to school at age six (we didn't have kindergarten in those days), I mainly remember family trips and a few other "not worth mentioning" things. It was exciting to be six and start to school. I had a sister five years older and a brother eighteen years older, my brother from an earlier marriage of my father. It is amazing how a six-year-old views life. However, I remember on the first day of school that I saw many mothers who looked so young. My mother produced me late in life, the last for our family. It was traumatic for me to see my mother with gray hair looking far older than the other kids' moms. My mother had begun to lose her hearing in her late teens, and by her late twenties was virtually deaf. By the time I came along (she was 35 years old), she was deaf. The deafness was probably not a factor because she lip-read beautifully. She always made sure she was one on one. She did not sign: that indicated disability—something less than perfect. As I think about it now, I realize it was my dad who thought my mother was beautiful and did not want her to be less than perfect, but it fit my mother's opinions concerning most matters to always be perfect. At any rate, I worried from that first day school began for me at age six whether or not she would be all right until I arrived back at home. Where the fear arose, I do not know. However, I know it was very real and long lasting.

School started with excitement for me, other than the trauma that my mother was older than other children's mothers. At the end of the first six weeks, I was rather proud of my straight-A report card. Straight A's had always been expected from and applauded for my older sister who was at that time in her sixth-grade year. She had all A's for the first five grades and her first six weeks in the sixth grade. As siblings usually operate, we were the same. Five years is a lot when children are vastly different in outlook and personality. We were that. At any rate, it became clear to me that my straight A was not as important as her straight A, and for some unrealistic reason, a problem child was born. From my earliest memory, I had been extremely shy for no known reason except that of a natural personality. Now I was a shy child who became a problem.

After the second six weeks began, my kitty was hit by a car and killed. That just didn't seem fair and produced great trauma although I said little about it after the day it happened. Fear for my mother dying became more of a problem. Day after day I became ill at school, and they called my mother to come get me. When she arrived, I felt safe and comforted. Because the illnesses were emotional, my stay at home was short from a lack of temperature, but soon after returning to school, I would throw up again, and the school-to-home cycle recurred. Unfortunately, I kept my fears to myself, telling no one about concern for my mother.

Eventually, I suppose reality set in, that school was a necessity. At that point, however, I did not want any part of it. I began to cause trouble at school. In my quiet way, I managed to pinch other children, pull pigtails, kick, shove, and generally make a complete nuisance of myself. When the teacher would ask me why I was misbehaving, I would say nothing. Generally, I shrugged my shoulders in answer to any question. When my parents asked why I was causing problems at school, I provided the same response. When it came to school, I was not communicative.

At the same time, I was doing no work at school. My grades were very poor. At first, being behind was chalked up to missing so many days. When they could not get me to consistently respond regardless of the punishment, everyone was at their wits' end. In our family, there had never been a problem like the one they faced with me. To say they were embarrassed is an understatement. As stated, failure or anything less than perfection was unacceptable. In our family, it was unheard of.

Grief set in with my parents. I will never know the pain they must have lived through. Today, memory of their grief saddens me greatly. They were highly respected members of our community. Although I never knew my maternal grandmother, who died before my birth, she and my grandfather were both college professors in the early 1900's when most people did not have a formal education. My mother's grandfather was a surgeon. Before losing her hearing, my mother was quite a musician. She was also valedictorian of her class in a large high school. A loser did not fit in the family.

Through it all, my parents were lovingly frustrated. They tried everything they knew. The problem was not short term either. Although I did become more accomplished with manipulating situations to make it appear that I was being mistreated at school, second grade and third grade came and went. One thing that did change for the most part after first grade was my picking on other children. However, along with not doing my schoolwork, I had learned to be destructive and deceptive. Third grade was especially difficult for everyone because my teacher had been a classmate of my mother's sister. Embarrassment for my family grew exponentially. Also, by this time, having produced little useful work, whatever good feelings I may have had about my ability two or three years before had vanished. They were moving me from grade to grade, however, because in those days, a teacher who had you in her class would most likely be required to try again with you the following year if you were not promoted. None of my teachers wanted to punish themselves for another year; thus, I was moved on.

Fourth grade appeared, at one point, to perhaps be a turnaround time for me. A student teacher was in the class for much of a nine-week period (perhaps she did not know my reputation as did the majority of the school personnel). My memory does not allow understanding how her magic worked on me. I only know everyone thought life was better, including me. Perhaps I must interject that my behavior was not that of class disturbance: I simply would not do my work. The devious things I did were unknown to my teachers, other students, and my parents. We always hear of kids in days gone by putting tacks in teachers' chairs, or other such things when the teacher was out. I did things of that nature. However, the missing link was that I did not do it to get other kids or the teacher's attention: I was a loner. No one knew who the culprit was. I did not want to be caught, and in all my years, I never was.

In my childhood, many schools had cloakrooms where coats, lunches, and storage items were kept. Because of my unwillingness to complete my work, I spent much of my time in the infamous cloakroom. It became a home away from home for me. I knew every square inch of each one. When I was in the fourth grade, however, there was a flaw in the structure. The room was formed with cinder blocks. I found that one had a crack, which was ever so slight and did not show. With days, or perhaps weeks of work, I managed to remove the block and replace it as often as I desired. It was not obvious that it could be removed unless you knew it was there. When it was removed from the rest of the wall, there was quite a cavernous space in which many things could be placed. However, most of those items could not be retrieved, once dropped into the "dark hole." One day I decided to place everyone's lunch there. It was certainly a mystery when lunchtime came, and all lunches had vanished. Mine was gone as well, of course, although it had been eaten before depositing its trash into the abyss! As I reflect on these memories now, they make me somewhat sick in a different way from the "sick" I was then.

Although the student teacher had a positive impact on me, it was too little and too short a time. I was convinced that I was stupid and the best thing for me to do was continue with my errant ways so no one would find out how stupid I really was. Fortunately, I thought, no one had told my parents about the IQ test results which I knew could not be good.

Fifth grade was probably the worst, behaviorally, but there is nothing new to report. Sixth grade was a different story. In my sixth grade year, my teacher was a man. He had been my sister's teacher when I started to school in the first grade. He loved my sister, and all of my family loved him. Now what would I do? How in the world I knew how to read and write I do not know. However, I managed to survive with mostly grades of B, as I remember. I had a really special boy friend as well. I had begun to be *very* fond of the opposite sex.

Unfortunately, with my shyness and feelings of inadequacy, moving into the seventh grade in a junior high school was frightening. My male teacher who had nurtured me almost daily the previous year was no longer there. In addition, there was a different teacher for every subject. It was just impossible. I was a late bloomer as well, so it was more than difficult when it was time for physical education class and a clothes change. At lunch, you were on your own. Everyone had someone to sit with. I always sat by myself, and I was uncomfortable. There were numerous boy friends, but boys and girls did not sit together in those days. I did not really want to sit with anyone else, but it was embarrassing to sit alone. Failure was my middle name.

School was not going well, so two months into the year, I faked an appendicitis attack. It was Halloween evening. The doctor was called, and I was carted off to the hospital. The doctor was perplexed. Although there were many things that just did not add up, any time the area over my appendix was touched, it was painful. (I didn't know that appendicitis usually hurts in mid-abdomen, so I said it hurt where the appendix was located.) Therefore, he believed it necessary to remove the appendix many days later, in the event he was missing something. I had been in the hospital for two weeks by the time it was removed.

Surgery was quite a relief. I was beginning to believe my illness ploy was not working. But, good results finally came. Recuperation would be six weeks. It had already been two weeks, and that would keep me safe from returning to school until after the Christmas holidays.

Much of that winter, like most winters before, I had swollen and sick tonsils. That *was* the truth. My parents had begun taking me to the doctor who had removed my appendix, and he suggested that with the history they provided relative to my constant sore throats, it might be wise to remove my tonsils in the spring. I thought, what a break! I wondered why I was being so fortunate, but considered myself very lucky indeed.

As a result of my many sore throats and bad tonsils, I was excused from physical education class for the year, and my tonsils were removed in the spring. I missed a lot more time. Actually, few of the teachers in junior high knew of my devious nature, and two came to see me at home and nurtured me along the way. My English teacher had my number as did the homemaking teacher, but at least two of the others were moved to look for some good. Although I missed the majority of the seventh grade, I moved on to eighth. It might be worth adding that I no longer attempted to entertain myself with devious activities at school. Again, the major complaint was that I wouldn't try. Also, I remained quite intent on boys. My interest was more as buddies than as boyfriends, but adults were unable to tell the difference. As time went by, however, the interest grew beyond buddies.

My sister married and moved to the northeast in late summer as my eighth-grade year began. Getting all the attention at home was wonderful. Also, there was a teacher who continued to encourage me along. I was extremely shy, but I was willing to talk with her some. Mostly, I just enjoyed being wherever she was. She allowed that without requiring me to make conversation.

Having missed so many years of learning, my grades were not wonderful, and my confidence was weak, but I made it through with B's and C's on my own. The standard around our house had not included B's, much less C's, but no one was complaining. My parents were not too excited that I spent a lot of time with boys, but it appeared to them that I might be doing a bit better. I was doing better in many respects. Unfortunately, I had become involved with other kids in my neighborhood who smoked cigarettes, and I was addicted as well. They are not to be blamed at all for my habit. I had begun to play with cigarettes many years earlier. In my elementary school years, I managed to steal cigarettes by the pack from my dad, hide them in my box camera, and smoke them alone. I was never caught at home, and never did I smoke a cigarette at school. Perhaps I feared detection. I certainly would have avoided my parents' suspicion at all costs. This was an area in which I did not want to disappoint them.

Ninth grade was at the same site as the seventh and eighth. I was the shortest person in my class. Over four hundred kids and I had to be the shortest. I was shy, short, and stupid. Lunch had continued to be difficult during the eighth grade, sitting alone. In the ninth grade, several girls from my church asked if I would like to sit with them. Although I had little to say, it was nice to feel less conspicuous at lunch. They were really wonderful people, no wild boys or cigarettes for them, and of course, they did not know about me. All they knew was that I attended the same large Baptist church as they. My daddy was a deacon, he taught a men's Sunday school class, and was otherwise very active in the church. Many of their parents were active as well. They seemed rather dull and boring to me, but I did recognize their worth. I think my parents were doing cartwheels in their hearts over my new friends at school. Of course, much of my time was spent with my old friends as well.

My grades improved, and I was now making A's and B's. How I learned anything over the course of my school career up to this point is nothing short of a miracle. When and how I really learned to read and write is a mystery. My reading comprehension was not very good, and had I understood that, I would have reread until I did comprehend. However, not having a clue, I continued thinking that I was stupid, but that I had everyone else fooled. Much of my life had been deception to this point; so, what was new? This time, deception was for a positive outcome. As I now look back, since credits begin accumulating at the ninth grade level, this was indeed a good time for me to move forward the best I could.

One of the young ladies with whom I was eating lunch each day lived half of the time with one set of grandparents and the other half with the other set of grandparents. Her dad's parents lived on the street directly behind us. In fact, the back of their property was directly behind our property. When we discovered this, she crawled through the back fence to visit (our lots were 210 feet deep, so it was some distance between the houses). During the visit, my friend and my mother entered a discussion. My mother asked a lot of questions about her family. It was found that Beth's mother, who died when Beth was two years old, had been in my mother's Sunday school class as a teenager. My mother was the type of person who was adored by everyone anyway, but for Beth, who loved the memory of her own mother, my mother was really special since she had taught her mother in Sunday school. A true friendship began. Beth was perhaps guarded because she had become somewhat aware of my wild side, but knowing my mother, allayed many fears.

Certainly, I did not fit in my family. My parents, however, were unaware of many of my shortcomings. After all, I had come a long way. Also, I had some wonderful girls with whom I kept company. My other friends remained as well for a short time. One day I was with one of the other friends on the way to get my dad from work. (It is probably fair for me to admit that this was not a bad kid; she was actually a good kid whom I had encouraged to smoke and get involved with a wrong crowd.) Yes, I had a driver's license now and kept the wheels warm. There were many needed trips for me to take, and going to get my dad was one of them. We left early, however, so we could go by the local drive-in and order a coke. We parked beside two guys who were older, but we thought, cute. I asked if either of them had a cigarette. One of the guys smoked, one did not. We were given cigarettes and traded phone numbers. Fortunately, they were decent young men. In those days, conversations at the local drive-in were common. Most of the time, from a crime standpoint, they were benign, but anything could have been possible. It was now around 1960.

The younger one who did not smoke, a nineteen year old, called me a few days later and came to our house. He was from a small town a few miles away. We had relatives in this town, and my dad checked him out and found him to be a nice young man who was a devout church member and from a good family. Although he was three years older at an age where that is quite a difference, my parents let me date him. They were in hopes that I would discontinue my relationship with the boy I was currently dating. Perhaps it was dangerous, but it worked. I did not stop smoking, but I did not smoke while I was with this young man. However, we did not date very long. The other guy who had been with him in the car at the first encounter began calling me, and we spent a great amount of time on the phone. My parents were reluctant to let me date him since he was twenty-four years old. He was very shy around my parents and unwilling to just "kick around at my house." Therefore, we spent hours on the phone. Eventually, I convinced my parents they should allow me to date him on a double date. I was now in the latter part of my tenth grade year, making acceptable grades, and generally shaping up. I continued eating lunch at school and socializing often with the group of about eight girls from church. We slept at each other's houses more than occasionally, usually as a group, but we paired up with different ones as best friends.

I continued to be closer with Beth than most of the other eight, although Sue later became my closest friend. Lee (the twenty-four year old young man) and I had double-dated with my friend from the neighborhood and a friend of Lee's who was a preacher's kid. For some reason, that made it okay with my parents for us to go. Lee was quite the gentleman although the preacher's kid was the wildest of the bunch! As time went by, my parents came to accept Lee and approved of our dating. Lee smoked and I continued to smoke. However, other than being a smoker (although my dad had started smoking when he was young as many others had in his era, he was opposed to my dating young men who smoked), there was nothing else about him my parents would have disapproved of. An unlikely, positive turn was taking place in my life. I thought my good grades were a fluke, that my intelligence was lacking, but life had improved. My time with the wrong crowd became less and less. Unfortunately, I had the cigarette habit and smoked on nights and weekends when I was on a date with Lee. My parents were still unaware.

By the eleventh and twelfth grades, my life was static with Lee, Sue, Jim, and Dan. Sue and Jim became an "item" when she and I were in the eleventh grade. They doubled with Lee and me most every weekend. During the twelfth grade, Sue and Dan became an "item." After graduation, they married. Lee and I discussed marriage, but my dad suggested that we wait one year. For one thing, I had been having health problems; for another, if it was good that we marry, it would be just as good a year later. Lee agreed to wait. By the way, I was still very shy with people I did not know well.

During my twelfth grade year, my deteriorating health became more serious, and I determined after graduation from high school not to go to college. I graduated magna-cum-laude but was convinced it was just by chance, although I did not share this opinion with anyone. Although my serious health condition was a factor, I used it as an excuse not to attend college. My grades had been good in high school, but being very shy and convinced that I would experience failure in college since I was not that smart, I decided to get a job. I got a job at an insurance company working with car policies and claims. Cars were and are a weakness for me. I have always had a love affair with automobiles.

LIFE GOES ON

Many tests were completed to determine what was wrong with my health. My diagnosis was leukemia. Several physicians were contacted, including two blood specialists. All produced the same diagnosis. My platelet count was very low, and I got a steady regimen of massive doses of steroids. My body responded poorly to steroids, so they were discontinued four months into treatment. I truly felt lousy. This was not a dreamed up illness on my part. At one point in the fall following graduation from high school, my condition worsened to the point that I was given only three months to live. In those days, physicians were not as open with their assessments as they are today. Often during those times, doctors did not give you dismal news, but my doctor told me there was concern that I would die soon. I was not all that concerned; after all, it would deliver me from all my problems. But I worried about my parents. By this time, I had grown to appreciate my parents greatly and realized the many sacrifices they had made for me throughout my life. Knowing it would be devastating for them, I asked the doctor not to tell them. He agreed. Unknown to me, however, he had given them the same news, and they asked that he not tell me. He agreed. Today, at a time when lawsuits are rampant, and physicians must operate differently, this would not happen. I can say that for my family and me, not knowing that the other had the bad news was good. Many days it was difficult to go to work, but I did find through my job that the concern that I was stupid was not valid. Also, three months became four, four five, and so on. The diagnosis must be incorrect. When I continued to live, it was determined that I had ITP (idiopathic thrombocytopenic purpura, which results in a low platelet count and bruising of unknown origin) rather than leukemia. Was it a miracle? Was it a coincidence? It makes one wonder, or does it?

When spring came, I felt somewhat better though tired most of the time, but I began thinking about attending college. It appeared I wasn't going to die any time soon, and just maybe I could succeed. They had really been pleased with my work at the insurance company. Of course, I thought that would not be as tough as college. I spoke with my supervisor at work, and she encouraged me to attend college. She told me I was more competent in my job than anyone she had previously supervised. Although not totally convinced, I decided to check it out for myself.

I left the insurance company in May to attend summer school. One of the girls with whom I had eaten lunch in high school attended a college near my home and she went with me to register for the courses. During that summer, I completed a year of history and a year of Bible, required at the Methodist school I chose. Having spent my life in the Baptist church, I was comfortable with my foundation for the Bible course. Summer ended, and I had accumulated four grades of B. This was not wonderful by my standards, but acceptable. Being shy, I never said a word in class, and it appeared it would be helpful to engage in conversation, at least ask questions. I could not.

Fall came, and it was time to register again. I continued to date Lee, but we were content not to marry. During registration, I planned to take courses required of all students to get them behind me. I had no idea what to major in. That could wait until later. One required course I wanted to put off as long as possible was speech. However, as I registered, I found roadblocks at every turn. Courses needed for freshmen were plentiful as long as it was math, history, or English. I had completed my history course, so that was not necessary. I signed up for English, algebra, biology, and physical education; eleven of the fourteen hours I was planning to take. Nothing would fit my schedule except speech. I went to a speech professor and told him of my dilemma: how I was petrified to speak with people, much less make a speech. (As I think back on it now, it took something beyond me to speak with a professor about my problem!) I was planning to take my required speech course during my senior year. The professor with whom I spoke was a wonderful Christian man. Angels appear in many forms; he was sent for me. I left his station scheduled to take speech. To say there was peace in my heart about it would not be totally true, but this man was great!

At the college I chose, freshmen took a battery of tests in an orientation course that lasted six weeks. During that time I was concerned about how I would manage all these standardized tests, but there was little pressure applied. You simply showed up for class and completed tests. There was no grade; its purpose was to provide the school with information. My anxiety was that I had been allowed to enter the school based on my good high-school grades. I had been unaware that these tests were required. If my intelligence was unacceptable, would I be kicked out? I supposed I would find out later.

All of the regular classes started out well. My speech professor was wonderful. During the very first class session, all students in the class were asked by the teacher to tell their name, where they went to high school including the city, what they thought they were planning to major in, and why they were taking this speech course at this particular time. I was sitting on the back row, and as he went from student to student, I heard nothing anyone said. I was too concerned about what I would say. We did not even have to stand beside our chairs, but I was totally petrified. Over and over in my mind I thought, "Sharon Byas (my maiden name), Polytechnic High School, Fort Worth, Texas, I don't know yet, and because I had to." When it finally became my turn, I got it out, botched and shaky, but over!

On this day and one or two more during the first few class meetings, the professor gave me special attention in front of the entire class. This made me feel good, but it also embarrassed me. It had been my strategy in all classes through school to be as invisible as possible. In this class I was anything but invisible. One day he told me how "beautiful you are in blue" in front of the class. That year's Miss Texas was in that class. Oh, how embarrassing! It was during that particular class period or one soon thereafter that a speech to instruct or inform was assigned. I madly searched books and magazines in an effort to find a subject on which to speak. In a magazine, I found a how-to for floral arranging. This was it. I would make several visuals on poster board depicting each step. I must do well. I did not at any cost want to let down my professor. As the day neared for me to present my speech, my anxiety became greater and greater. I had practiced it alone at home more times than could be counted, but I was scared! We drew numbers to determine the order in which speeches were to be given. When my number came up, I went to the podium with all of my visuals, shaking, but as confident as I could be under the circumstances. However, as I began, everything went south. My knees knocked, my mouth became dry, and even with my visuals and unnumbered practice trials, the speech was terrible. I wanted to hurry and get back to my seat. My three-minute speech (the time was correct) was over. Embarrassed and disappointed, but what a relief that it was over!

As with each speech, the professor went to the front of the room to critique. Oh dear, more torture to come. His first words were, "Sharon, you hate floral arranging. Why did you choose it as your topic?" He said these words in such a way that the tension in the room was splattered, just like a drop of water in slow motion. At that point, words came that it was the only thing I could find, but that he was certainly correct, floral arranging was somewhere near the bottom on my list of interests. The critique continued, but my anxiety for the moment was gone. Furthermore, for some reason, the rest of the students in class were very kind and even gave me some positive strokes.

The professor invited me to visit with him in his office, and I went to see him the following day. He took a great deal of time getting to know me. This began a friendship that lasted long after college, until his death. After many conferences with him during that first fall semester in college, I found that my IQ was above 130 (he had looked at my file and checked me out). It was hard for me to believe, so he received permission from the college dean to show me my scores. Wow, it was true! All the years I thought myself stupid and not capable of success had indeed affected my reading comprehension, but even that was continuously improving. Within a short period of time, I was on par with the best, unless I was experiencing anxiety. Even today, when I am experiencing great anxiety and the subject matter is complicated, I often have to read something twice to get it. I am told that is normal, but my expectation throughout life has been otherwise.

In this book, I will not review each speech from that first semester, but know that I received in excess of thirty college hours in speech by graduation, giving me a triple major. Originally, I declared my major as pre-med. and took many courses in biology, anatomy and physiology, genetics, and other related subjects. However, my health, although not like it had been previously, continued to be a problem. I was tired much of the time and my platelet count was very low. Although an elective spleenectomy was performed and my energy level improved, I was encouraged to leave medicine to others. Medical school would simply be too rigorous.

This was not good news for me. At the time, I had my heart set on being a surgeon. As it turned out, I could have kept any schedule, but not seeing into the future, I wondered what else there was for me to do? Some might think the logical move would be to nursing, but that was definitely not for me. I had wanted to be a surgeon. Surgeons visit with patients who have a referral from another physician. The surgeon determines if surgery is necessary and takes care of it when needed. Conversing with someone about how they felt or taking vital signs had zero interest for me except as a necessary adjunct to my surgical practice. Nursing was definitely out!

There was teaching, but my public school memories were not particularly good, and I certainly did not want to teach speech. If I did decide to teach, I wanted two teaching fields. Making detailed speeches had become something I did relatively well; however, impromptu speaking was still not my thing. Shyness had not left me. So, with all the science I had taken, biology was one field, and the speech professor encouraged me to take physical education as well, for two reasons. Many science courses doubled for physical education (physiology, tests and measurements, health, and others), and he said I looked like an athlete. Think of it: a person who had not wanted to change clothes at school, with physical education as one of her majors! As mentioned earlier, I was excused from physical education in junior high school because I kept talking the doctor into long-term excuses. In high school, with my blood problems, I was excused most of the time as well. I had *no* previous experience.

Fortunately, I did have some physical ability, although many physical education classes are "study and test" rather than "do."

Contrary to the opinion many have that it is a no-brainer subject, there is a great deal of brainwork involved. Tests and measurements courses, in addition to a host of others, are filled with mathematical equations, trigonometry, biological principles of muscle movement, and physics. Perhaps this is the subject where those who can, do, and those who can't, teach. Some who can do, also teach.

During the same period of time, two tragic events occurred in my life. I had surgery, and five months later, my grandfather on my mother's side with whom I had at one time been very close, died. It was a year prior to graduation, but with all I had going at school, it did not settle in to the degree it did after graduation. (I will explain this in a later chapter.) When the event occurred, I had what they called a nervous breakdown. The phobias I had for so many years about mother's death were not completely gone, but they had been replaced by a deep love for her. When I was younger, I was close with my dad. By this time, I was very close with both parents. I adored my mother. I never wanted her to hurt in any way. When she hurt, I hurt. She loved her papa very much, and her grief broke my heart. My grandfather had died at a family reunion that my mother had wanted to attend, but I used a lame excuse that I had too much college work to do and could not go. Daddy wouldn't go without me, so we did not go.

Although we only lived three doors down from my granddad, prior to his death I had avoided his coming to visit since my surgery four months earlier (my spleen had been removed to improve my blood problem). I had asked my daddy to tell him I was too tired every time he came to see me. He was talkative, and I was still recuperating. When he died, my guilt overwhelmed me. I did not have adequate coping skills for a family death. I was 21 years old, and he was my first loss. I had a kitty cat that I was *very* attached to, as well, who died a week or so after my grandfather's death. The death of the cat was actually the last straw. As a result, my physician prescribed medications for my depression, uppers and downers to get me through the day. At school, I functioned relatively well. It was at home that I had problems. The old fear of my mother dying came back in full force. As was my usual pattern, I told no one. Pills got me through. The year and a half to reach graduation was difficult. My major had to be changed. I was not happy about my new plan for my life's work, and my surgery had not gone well. My grandfather and my pet had died. I worried about my mother. It was simply more than I could handle.

WORK AND MARRIAGE

When I graduated from college, the next step was to get a job. I procrastinated. Physically, I felt well. However, psychologically I was in shambles. Thus, my physician prescribed more pills. It was indeed time to flood school districts with applications for a teaching job. I did not. Near the end of the summer, my dad spoke with a school board member in our church and mentioned my needing a job. Our city had a large school district, and two days later I received a call from the personnel department requesting information about my teaching fields. I provided the information, and they sent me an application through the mail. I completed the forms and mailed them back. It was almost time for school to begin the fall semester. A call came a few days later telling me that there were no biology openings, but there was an opening in elementary physical education. I accepted.

The first day began. It was almost like the first day for me in elementary school when I saw that my mother looked so much older than other mothers did. There were probably more than sixty elementary schools in this city, and I was assigned the same school I had attended as a child! The school had been remodeled since I was a student. The first thing I had to do was check to see if the loose cinder block in the infamous cloakroom was still there. It brought back many memories. Also, they were not using the third floor of the old building except for storage. Since it was the first year for physical education at elementary schools in this district, and no other space was available, the third floor became my office. It was not a really large area, but when weather was extremely inclement, there were times I took the kids up there as well. My class sizes were anywhere from 50 to 143. Those days are certainly unlike today!

As I looked through the storage area from day to day in that third floor space during my conference period, I found many old books from my early days. There were *Dick and Jane* books galore. I remembered the covers on many books. Being on heavy medication already (not obvious to others), and having a dreadful phobia, fearing for my mother's death, it became very difficult to go to work each day. All I wanted to do was sleep. Also, I hated my work, and hate is a very accurate word for my feelings. Indeed, my problems were far more numerous than concern for my mother, but I was not aware that my depression had more than one contributing factor. I did not confide in anyone and never saw a psychiatrist or any doctor other than my general practitioner who knew I needed something to get me through whatever I was experiencing.

During that first year of teaching, my friend Beth, who had met and fallen in love with someone while in college, married. She asked me to be in her wedding party. Her husband-to-be had a brother who was a teacher in a nearby school district and was a photographer on the side. He took pictures at the wedding, and I met him there. Although I was quasi engaged to Lee at the time, after Beth's new husband's brother called on numerous occasions to ask for a date, I decided to go so he would leave me alone! It was now April first (only foolish for him). I wanted to get this date and the school year behind me. The school year was nearing a close, and I was barely surviving psychologically.

On the evening of April first, we went out. This was one great guy. He was everything any girl could ever want. He was nice looking, well mannered and wonderful in every way. He didn't drink, smoke, curse, or do any of the things I had been reared to believe wrong. Should I let this one get away? I didn't drink or curse; I still smoked although I did not let him know at the time. At first I even attempted to quit, but it just did not seem to happen; I kept starting back. We had dated only a couple of months when he asked me to marry him. At that time, I confessed about my smoking habit and that I would like to quit but was not being successful. I additionally told him about my taking prescription drugs for depression. His response was that it would be healthier for me not to smoke, but it would not affect whether or not he loved me. Additionally, whatever my doctor thought I needed to take was all right with him. I decided marriage would be a good thing for me. This was a great guy, and I really cared a lot for him. This perhaps was what I was missing.

Summer arrived, and I began work on my master's degree at a university about thirty-five miles or so from home, and I decided to live in the dorm so I could be alone. My fiancé came to see me more often than I would have liked. This should have put up a red flag, but I gave it little thought. When he came, we talked about our marriage and planned to wed during the Thanksgiving holidays. There was a lot to plan and do. My mother, however, was just the right person to plan a wedding. Although I had finished college and worked, I was shy and had no interest in things like weddings. It would have been better in my view to elope, but neither my husband-to-be nor my mother would have agreed. What my mother thought or wanted was very important to me.

In addition to planning my wedding, two other events occurred that summer. My mother's sister, with whom she was extremely close, died, and I changed school districts. My aunt's death did not affect me to the same degree my grandfather's had although it created some sorrow, of course. My mother was truly struck with grief. She did not talk about it a great deal, but she would sit alone in our back room or take extended walks in the yard. She had not exhibited this behavior before. I never gave it a thought at the time, but she also had her last child getting married in five months, the wedding to plan (this would have been fun for her in better times), and this troubled child would be leaving home. As an adult, I have often thought about the grief I caused my parents as a brat child, but I did not give adequate credence to the pain they suffered after the childhood misbehavior left, and more serious concerns arose including my physical and psychological health. The fact that I was a smoker would have been grief enough for my mother. Knowing that, you can imagine how much grief everything else caused. At the same time, my mother suffered for her other daughter and the grandchildren who lived two thousand miles away.

As stated, the other momentous thing to occur that summer was that I changed school districts. I had one year of dreadful experience behind me. Also, as it turned out, it was late in the summer again before I decided to change jobs. As before, I did not initiate an interview with the new district. My husband-to-be spoke with the personnel director who informed him there were no biology openings available, but there was an elementary physical education position open. Not again! It was disappointing not to teach biology, but I wanted to change districts.

As the school year began, I remained on anti-depressants although the dosage was somewhat less than previously. It was exciting to re-decorate the house in which my intended lived. There was a lot of painting and other renovating to be done, and I spent endless hours working toward completion by the wedding date. Also, I truly liked the school I was teaching in. There were many wonderful teachers, and I particularly liked the principal and school secretary. Life was getting better, although I was not totally sure about marriage. I truly loved my guy, but somehow marriage was a step I was not really prepared for. As the wedding day neared, I had some doubts but suspected that that was the way it was with everyone. After all, I was 24 years old; it was time to marry.

We finished getting the house ready for a new occupant, and my mother had everything lined up for the wedding. As the day neared, I became more anxious, but to make mention of that would not have been something I would do. After all, I was marrying a wonderful man, one who loved me dearly and would do whatever it took to make my life the best possible.

Our wedding day arrived, and I received a dozen long-stemmed red roses. The hour came to get to the church. My anxiety continued to grow. Interestingly, just as I was getting ready to go down the aisle on my dad's arm, my sister-in-law asked if I was sure this was what I wanted to do. How could she have picked up on my feelings when no one else had? I think I told her it was too late. This was an expensive church wedding, and not only had my mother worked very hard to get everything just right for the event, it was quite a stretch on the family budget to make it happen. I could not change my mind now; the pain and embarrassment would be far greater than I could bear. What would I do if I didn't marry now? This was a great guy; I needed to get my head on straight.

As soon as the wedding was over, we flew to New Orleans. The school district had given us three free days' absence, in addition to the Thanksgiving holidays, for our honeymoon. Such generosity— it was and is greatly appreciated. New Orleans was fun. We spent most of our honeymoon buying Christmas presents for our families since it was only a month away. I had married a wonderful person who truly loved me. What more could any girl want?

We returned home after our honeymoon and started what would be considered a normal life. Work continued, and I really liked the people with whom I worked. I became friends with one of the fifth grade teachers. I invited her and her husband to our house for dinner and to play cards. We had a good time, and this began a great friendship. Most weekends, we were at one or the other's home socializing. It is true that I was not shy with this couple after I got to know them. We had drinks from time to time as we socialized. This was not something I had done much of previously, but we actually drank very little. My husband did not like alcohol, and that probably kept me from being too exposed as well.

The school year ended, and I was offered a biology assignment. Science had certainly been the subject I intended to teach, so it was surprising even to me, but I did not want to leave the elementary school where I was. The regimentation of physical education was in keeping with my personality, and I felt like I fit in at my current school. I turned it down and stayed one more year.

During that year, it was common for someone to ask if my head was stopped up. My answer always was that I was fine. I was questioned so often about my resonance that I asked my doctor if there might be a problem. He examined my sinuses and suspected I was experiencing sinus trouble, but he suggested I see a specialist. When I met with the specialist, he found adenoidal tissue that needed to be removed. Soon thereafter, surgery was performed to remove the tissue. It was uneventful, and I was quickly back to my regular schedule. No longer did anyone ask if I had a cold or some other problem that would cause me to sound funny. It was found that I had a severe allergy to the developer used to process photographs, and it was believed to have possibly been the culprit that caused the tissue to grow.

My husband had been involved with photography for many years. In the Marine Corps he had taken pictures. Where he now taught biology, he took pictures for the school annual. He truly enjoyed photography and took wedding pictures after hours as well. He worked with students before and after school to teach them how to take good, balanced pictures. The school district began a class in photography for students to take as an elective, and my husband was asked to be the teacher. At first he taught both biology and photography, but as interest in photography grew, he was teaching photography the entire day. Now it had been determined that a critical component of his teaching was causing me to be ill. The developer is a strong acid, and the smell gets into clothes, hair follicles, etc. Therefore, it became necessary for him to take an extra change of clothes with him to work, then shower and wash his hair before returning home. He never once complained. This was one jewel of a man! At the end of the year, he asked to teach biology again. It truly broke my heart because I knew how very much he loved photography but I had no other solution.

After having spent three years teaching elementary physical education (one year was in another district), I decided I was ready to change to science. Classroom teaching was quite a change from physical education and the outdoors. Also, I missed my friends at the elementary school, but I found that I did prefer to work with older kids. The elementary age had been fine to regiment, but the older age was far better for me from a liking standpoint. Life and work did not seem to have that many joys, and teaching was not particularly fulfilling, but life went on. After all, what was life supposed to be? You got married, had children, worked, and lived. Although I did not feel maternal, I did attempt to have children, but that was not to be. Although I was able to get pregnant, I was unable to carry to term.

In addition to our teaching jobs, my husband and I had gotten involved with a motivational group and pyramid scheme. We had no idea it was frowned upon. It had been really good for us, both individually and as a couple. However, the government came down hard on pyramid schemes, and the company was broken up into sales groups. My husband got the opportunity to go to California with a company selling stainless-steel cookware. We discussed what seemed to be a good thing. All of the motivational activity had provided us with a family of friends. We were mesmerized and did not want to give it up.

Wow! We sold our house in one week, both quit our teaching jobs, and moved to California. It was hard for me to leave home, but I did not really like working either. Also, it appeared to me that my husband really wanted to go. After all, he had given up enough for me that this should be a simple thing to do. So, late in the second year of my teaching science, I left my job before the school year had ended, and we moved to California. Before I left, I asked my principal about going. I was concerned about breaking my contract. He assured me that it might be difficult for my husband to find a teaching job after breaking his contract without cause, but it was acceptable for a wife to break a contract to move with her husband. I called the central office and got the same reply.

Chapter 6

CALIFORNIA/DIVORCE/ MARRIAGE

Off we went to California, but not long after we arrived, we were disenchanted with the company. My husband became aware of another person who had quit to start his own business. Silkscreen printing on T-shirts had become big business in California as a new venue for advertising. Photography skills were important in this business. Therefore, my husband began to spend many hours with his acquaintance, learning new skills. The chemicals I had been allergic to were not used in the silk-screen process, therefore allowing a new possibility.

California was not an answer to my depression. Day after day I hoped would be my last. We often discussed my disappointment; however, we had little money, and no jobs back home. Neither of us really wanted to teach at that point, and he was truly interested in his new business. After we had been there awhile, I began to mention home more and more. He said he wanted to return home as well, and we would as soon as he felt comfortable that his knowledge base was sufficient to start his own business in Texas. I wrote my mother every day, something very unusual for me.

One morning about 2 A.M., I rolled over in bed and said I would really be glad when we could go home. He said, "How about now?" We got out of bed and were finished packing by four-thirty that morning and on the road. We didn't drive long until we were too tired to continue. We stopped at a hotel for a few hours, then continued our trip. We drove until we arrived home. It was about four in the morning, and neither of us wanted to disturb our parents, so we called some friends and woke them up. We went to their house and talked with them until late morning. We then called my parents and told them we were home. Home with eighty-eight dollars in the world. We had spent the equity from the house and the remaining money we had. Here we were—no money, no jobs, but home.

We stayed with my parents for six weeks, then his for six weeks. My dad gave us half his garage to use for the silk-screening business. Since there was no money, my husband went out and secured orders with fifty percent down so he could buy the materials to produce the product. He made a makeshift printer on which to silkscreen the shirts. He could build anything with his hands and was quite an artist as well as photographer; just what was needed for this business. After the twelve weeks with our parents, there was sufficient money to lease our own house. It was my job to help print, hang to dry (we did not have a T-shirt dryer yet), package, and help prepare for delivery. I often accompanied my husband on deliveries, but I delivered little alone. In my mid-twenties, I had developed a phobia that made it difficult for me to drive on the freeway alone. Depression, phobias, and a lack of zest for life continued to surround me.

After less than a year, we bought a nice house in a good neighborhood. My husband used the garage and several rooms for different business needs. There were enough orders that it became necessary to buy several pieces of expensive equipment to keep up with customer demand. When we had returned to Texas, silk-screen advertising on T-shirts was very new. Our business was one of the first of its kind, and customers were willing to accept one or two-color printing. As other competitors came along, it was necessary to offer a greater variety; thus, the additional equipment was needed.

Therefore, I thought it best that I get a job outside the business to generate money. I interviewed at a popular hamburger chain because managers at this company made really good money. I found after I was hired that I was the first woman hired directly into management in the Texas region. I liked that information!

The work involved many long hours. One week, I punched a clock just to see how many hours I spent there. The verdict was ninety that week. Many weeks I worked less than that, but eighty plus would have been a good average. I took great pride in my work, and the competition of those days among managers provided a thriving life for me. The money provided everything we needed and more. Additionally, my depression, phobias, and general malaise improved.

About two years after my getting the new job, our equipment was paid for. I had been transferred more than five times at work. Every time a store needed a fireman, I was sent. Each time, I was honored and given another good raise in pay, but it was hard on the body. We decided I would quit and take a break.

Unfortunately, the depression became far worse after I left my job to work at home. It was more and more difficult for me to get up each day. My husband was the most understanding and loving man in the world, but I decided to leave and go home to my parents.

Soon thereafter, I filed for divorce. I got a job at a steel-forging company as a bookkeeper. The money was good, and I got an apartment. Soon I became comptroller and treasurer of the board of the corporation where I worked. I spoke with my ex often, and only five months after the divorce was final, I decided I had made a horrible mistake by getting a divorce. This wonderful man still wanted to be my husband, so we remarried.

We had been married over seven years when we got the divorce, and we remarried two months prior to the original eight-year anniversary. We celebrated anniversaries on the original date. He continued with his silk-screen business, and I continued to work with the forging company.

About six months after we re-married, I realized it had been a mistake. At this time, I did not mention it to my husband, family, or friends. I thought I would just try to keep on plugging. We built a new, even larger home and I tried to settle in.

For more than another year, I continued with the forging company. A local CPA had provided me with sufficient knowledge to file quarterly taxes for the corporation, and I was completing monthly profit and loss statements, but I was not as comfortable with my accounting knowledge as I thought was necessary. The forging business was doing well, but I was always concerned that I might make a mistake that would be disastrous for the corporation. Both the owners and CPA tried to encourage me, but with my "I must know and understand everything" attitude, I felt inadequate. At the same time, my husband and I were doing well financially. We had bought a new house, new vehicles, had money in the bank, and life by all appearances was excellent.

Not only had I been concerned that my accounting knowledge was not adequate, there was something in me that wanted to give the classroom another try. I had changed a great deal since my last teaching job, and I was, after all, educated to be a teacher. I discussed how I felt with my husband. Since I was the one who handled all the finances, he suggested that I should be the one who determined whether or not we could afford for me to take this huge cut in salary. We had very few bills except our house payment (his business was in another part of town in a rented building and was self sustaining). My good paying jobs had provided for our wants as well as necessities.

As I began to seek a teaching job, I found that doors did not open. I went to two different school districts and did not get a job. One told me that money was tight. My master's degree and five years experience placed me on a scale considerably above a beginner. Therefore, beginners and near beginners were sought to save taxpayer dollars. This did not seem realistic to me, but it was what I was told. I decided to call a friend who was a principal in the school district I left five years earlier, and I asked him to look through my file to see if there was anything awry. He informed me that I had a "do not rehire" on my file. With the passage of five years, he was unable to ascertain who had placed it there. All other information was glowing, including appraisals and other comments. Glowing comments and a "do not rehire" did not really compute. This saddened me. Although I had many personal problems, I had been a good employee and adequate teacher. Students had liked me and believed me to be a good and caring educator. This was what I thought was desirable.

Summer was almost over, but I did not give up. One day on my lunch hour at the forging company, I went to the school administration building in the city where my current job was located. I had not considered a teaching job there; it was about twenty-five miles from my home. The two districts where I was turned down were closer to my house. I went in, asked for directions to the personnel office, filled out an application, and spoke with the personnel director. It just happened that the personnel director was leaving for his lunch. He spoke with me as I stood in the outer office, then invited me to speak with him at that time. I went into his office and told him my saga, including how I had left my teaching job on a whim five years earlier and moved to California. I told him how it had been such a mistake to break my contract, but it was so, whether

I liked it or not. I would have waited two months and then joined my husband in California had I been told it was the thing to do. I told him if he would give me a job, I would work for the pay of a bachelor's degree with no experience. He informed me that if I were hired, I would receive my scheduled pay.

As it turned out, again there were no biology openings, but an opening at a middle school for eighth-grade science, which was a combination of earth and life science, was available. I did not know anything about geology, meteorology, oceanography, or other earth studies, but I certainly was knowledgeable about the biology half of the assignment. I was willing to take other courses or whatever was necessary to get the assignment. Texas law allowed me to teach the classes without specific courses in earth science because I had many varied science studies. So the personnel director sent me to meet the principal of the school where the opening was. We hit it off immediately, and he requested for me to be hired.

Amazed, I went back to work and gave a two-week notice. It was three weeks until school would start. I had a week to prepare for my teaching assignment. Both psychologically and physically, I felt healthier than anytime in many, many years. I remained very shy, but it had not been difficult to talk with either the personnel director or the school principal, and it was extremely important to me to really do a good job. I asked for books early and began preparing lesson plans. Somehow, I was not disappointed that a high school biology job was not available. I was not only grateful to have this job, I was thrilled with the new principal. I truly liked him.

TEACHING AGAIN

The first day arrived for teachers, and I was there early. When I drove up, another lady was arriving. She spoke to me and started a conversation. Although I would have never started a conversation, and in all probability would not have spoken, I did respond. It was her first day in the school district as well. She was going to teach reading and homemaking. She had previous experience in another school district as did I.

It was a very large middle school, having in excess of eighteen hundred students. The school was clean and well organized. I liked the location of my classroom and the teacher next door who was several years older than I, and had taught science for some time. Her background was in geology with a wealth of knowledge that went with it. What a break that was for me! She and her husband were retired marines. Her husband had been a colonel in the Marine Corps and was now a physics teacher at the high school next to our middle school. She was a regimented person as was I. Although I enjoyed the kids more than I think she did, and although we did not always agree on the way things should be done, it was extremely helpful to have her wealth of earth-science knowledge next door. Actually, I liked this lady very much, and the three years I spent teaching science next door to her were truly good years.

It was obvious to all that I had a way with kids, even those who caused problems. I spent a lot of time before school meeting with any student who desired. Many of those who wanted to spend time with me before school were ones who did not fit for some reason or another. They were either having problems at home with their parents, their parents were divorcing, or they didn't have friends to meet with as they waited for school to begin each day. I allowed them to sit around and talk with one another, or if desired, to talk with me. Often, one would seek me out to tell me about a problem and ask me for my opinion. At times, groups would want to talk with me about things that were on their minds. My group of kids expanded as time went by and included many in students as well.

After completing my first year at this school, the principal decided to schedule a plethora of problem students in my classes for the following year. It was true, I had a real love for these kids, but through attempting to work with them in droves, I was totally stressed. Some of the students in my classes were learning disabled, which was the reason for their behavior problems, and some were psychologically disabled, with an inability to keep still. With thirty or more students in each class, it was difficult to keep my sanity. Even with considerably smaller numbers, I do not think I would have been capable of really doing an adequate teaching job. Since I had a wonderful relationship with the principal, I discussed my concerns after a while. He acknowledged that they had never tried to place so many problem kids in anyone's classes before, but it appeared if there was hope for them, I might be the one to unlock the key.

He told me he decided to put them in my classes as a result of several incidents that had occurred the previous year. One incident involved a truly difficult, large-for-his-age thirteen year old who had been in a fight with another student. It concerned me that several teachers were watching them fight in the hallway, not intruding to avoid being hurt. Two of the teachers were men, who I felt should have jumped in, but they did not. Therefore, I did. In order to avoid injury to myself, I pushed the boys with great force to separate them. As I provided the push, the larger boy hit his face on a locker, bloodying his nose. Although I believed I had done the right thing, I was concerned that his parents might decide to sue the school district. This was new back then—not much thought had been given to lawsuits in school districts, but I had come from the business world where there were constant concerns. I spoke with the principal, who was extremely supportive, and said he was pleased with my actions and that I would be supported completely.

After worrying for two days, the young man I had pushed into the locker came to my room before school. His mother wasn't with him, so how did he get into the school? He was supposed to be in trouble for his fight. As I walked out into the hall to speak with him, I shut my classroom door (several students were in my room as usual before school), and he said he wanted to apologize for his behavior two days before. He said he had sneaked up to my room to tell me. I told him it was necessary that I take him to the office since he was there without permission. He said he realized that, but he wanted to get to me first even if he got into more trouble for sneaking in. We went to the office, and I talked with the principal. The student had been suspended for three days for the fight, so he had to be sent home. Before he left to return home, he asked if he might be transferred into my class when his suspension was over. He said no one had ever stopped one of his fights before, and he thought I was cool. Even though I wondered if he had an ulterior motive, I said it would be fine. As it turned out at the end of the year, he did not pass the course, but his overall school behavior had greatly improved.

It was as a result of this incident and others the previous year, that I was given a rather rugged schedule. Another incident stands out that occurred during the second year (the year I had so many problem kids). One of the problem kids whom I had really gotten attached to burst through one of the large glass doors after school one Friday. Naturally the glass broke, and he had a large gash in his back. It was bleeding profusely. We were unable to get hold of a parent or any relative. It was critical that something be done. The butterfly bandages just wouldn't hold. What should I do, risk a suit or risk death? I really cared for this kid, so the answer was simple. I secured needle, thread, and alcohol. Over an hour passed before we were able to contact a family member. I was certainly relieved when they took him to the hospital and although my handiwork was rugged, it was praised. This incident became known all through the school and actually brought accolades from students as well as adults. When his back healed, his behavior began to improve. Unfortunately, after graduating from high school where he had become an average student, he was at the wrong place at the wrong time, was thought to be someone else, was shot, and died. It really hurt me when he was killed; I had been so excited when he changed his ways. It pleases me, however, that he died knowing he was a capable and worthy person.

During the following year, my third at the school, I was given the best schedule anyone could possibly want. The principal made sure there were no problem kids in any of my classes! I will always look back on that year as a perfect year. I continued to counsel the kids who loved and needed me before school, and I also had those everyone would love in the classroom. It was truly the best of both worlds.

In the middle of that wonderful year, my principal asked me if I had ever considered school administration. With my business background, organizational skills, and way with kids, he believed it would be something to think about. I told him I had not considered anything other than the classroom and was happy where I was.

Teaching had indeed been different these past three years. Life was very good! I was truly happy for the first time in many years. I had greatly curtailed my smoking two or three years before, although I had not completely stopped (I was not willing to take a chance that students might smell cigarettes on my breath or clothes, so I did not smoke until after school each day). I needed fewer drugs to feel normal. Also, I had become friends with the person I met on the first day of school two and a half years earlier. She was divorced with three sons. The sons had originally lived with her, but one by one as they aged, they had gone back to live with their dad. My new friend and I began to go many places together over the period of the previous year. I had a science club, and I took these students on weekend field trips. My friend went with us. She was so much fun to be with. It was really nice to have a wonderful friend.

It became more and more difficult to be married. My husband was a great guy, but for some reason, I was anxious and depressed when I was at home. It was indeed difficult to admit failure a second time. Although I had realized almost as soon as we remarried that it was the wrong thing to have done, I had decided to keep the 'til death do us part promise.

After Christmas the third year after my return to teaching, I asked for a divorce. My husband moved into the building where he had his business. This divorce was very difficult to go through. It may be hard for the reader to believe I really cared for my husband, but I truly loved him and always will. It was hard for him to accept, and he decided to fight me. When we got the first divorce, I had left with nothing. Perhaps he expected the same this time.

We went through a bitter divorce that took about two years, including all appeals. We had accumulated a lot of things, and we fought over who got what! The fact that he became a fighter helped me move on. It simply was not right, in my mind, for him to get everything just because I was the one who wanted the divorce. It additionally angered me that he attempted to use my friendship with another woman in a damaging and negative way during the proceedings. My wonderful parents and a special cousin attended the trial, providing great support for me. Although the divorce proceedings were difficult, I had been drug free with no pills and no cigarettes for some months. I had been a slave to drugs for about fifteen years. After two appeals on his part, we ended up in a trial without jury, and a judge decided the division of property. There was a possibility of one more appeal, but he let it stand. I was extremely grateful when it ended.

Chapter 8

ADMINISTRATION

During the divorce, I was in the process of changing jobs and moving into administration. My principal had continued to discuss his desire for me to be an assistant principal. He had been informed that he would be allowed an additional assistant the following year (that would make three), and he wanted me. I truly cared for my principal, and he had convinced me that I would make a wonderful administrator. Additionally, I had a way with kids in trouble. I was very strict but very caring. I did not tell anyone about my divorce being in progress and made plans to take college courses needed to move into administration. When I had gotten my masters degree, I had not considered administration; therefore, many courses were needed to secure the necessary certification. Numerous classes could be used to get a doctorate since I already had a master's degree. That was not important to me at the time; all I wanted was to get certified to be an administrator. It was acceptable to the state for you to complete courses while working as an administrator as long as you took a certain number each year until completion. Therefore, I took four courses in administration during summer school to get started, and one course each semester during the full-year term. It took me three years to complete.

My assignment did not turn out as I had planned. A new middle school (grades six through eight) was being built. There were three openings for assistant principals that year, one at the school where I taught, the new school, and a high school. My principal had requested that I be assigned with him, but I was not placed there. I was assigned to the new school. I was most disappointed because I wanted to be with the principal I cared so much about. He informed me that they would not assign me to him because the new school would have only one assistant, and it was believed that I was the best candidate to have that job. It did feed my ego. Both of the other positions had additional assistants to help carry the load, but it was not comforting to know that I was not the requested one for the job where I was assigned. The principal of the school where I was assigned had requested a male. Was it because he wanted the other person or because he was male? I did not know whether or not my being female would be of concern. Assistant principals were the disciplinarians; would he think a woman incapable of handling the really problem kids? It was a first in the school district to have a female as the only assistant principal in a secondary school. How would she handle it?

The principal was three years from retirement. He had been a principal for many years and had the reputation for being the toughest on students of any principal in the district. He was also very knowledgeable with both curriculum and school administration. During the summer, before I was on the payroll for an administrator, I was working on scheduling students every spare minute I had away from my college courses. I found that schedules do not simply fall into place. There is quite a system for assigning students into secondary classes. Today, computers are used for the purpose of scheduling, and they are certainly faster. However, because there are so many variables in scheduling because of the individual needs of students, it remains more accurate to schedule by hand.

Certainly, no one would go back to hand scheduling today; however, it remains the most student friendly although laborious.

By the time school began, the principal and I had become well acquainted, having spent several hundred hours working together through the summer. I was eager to be the best assistant principal there had ever been. I wanted our school to be the best school known to man as well. It was obvious I was willing to work around the clock to do a good job. Before school began, I had a lift because the principal told me he had made a mistake in requesting the other person. He said he thought I was going to be the best assistant he had ever worked with. This truly thrilled me since he had had numerous assistants through the years.

What a teacher this man was! He not only knew how to run a school, he knew how to teach someone to run a school. Although he knew everything that went on, he stayed out of my way until asked for help or an opinion. He handled the teachers; I handled the kids. He liked the way I disciplined students because I was strict. There was no question that I cared for the well-being of all kids. Most students knew I cared for them and wanted them to be whole people, but a good education was necessary at the same time. The principal and I were of like minds in the behavior department. It was impossible for learning to take place if there was disruption. Of course, this made teachers happy and the cycle of happiness was continuous. This was wonderful but unusual in the education business. Nearly all of us were happy, even students. When sent to the office for misbehavior, much of the time kids were apologetic and accepted punishment without complaining of unfair treatment.

It was difficult being the bad guy all the time. Each student I disciplined was always spoken to about their misbehavior, why consequences must occur, and what they might do in the future to avoid being in trouble. Students knew the consequence of their misbehavior. Both the principal and I were believers in corporal punishment and had provided a list of general infractions and their consequences, well known throughout the school. It remains my opinion that sparing the rod indeed is a poor choice in rearing a child. For some reason, we humans do not like physical pain. When pain is going to be inflicted, we often have an open mind for listening to how we might avoid this pain in the future. This is particularly true when it is being discussed with someone we know cares about us. We all need limits set and followed through. One of the major reasons we have difficulty providing certified teachers in the classroom today is the lack of discipline in schools. People with teaching degrees want to teach, not be wardens for kids whose parents think what they may have done should not be of any consequence. Over the years we have curtailed corporal punishment, and classroom discipline has consistently deteriorated. It was decided along the way that little psyches were damaged by violence (to paddle is violent, they say). It makes me wonder why we have such a population of senior citizens who experienced paddling and appear to be psychologically sound. School districts have yielded to the pressure as a result of threats for a lawsuit and lack of school-board support. School-board members have political positions. After all, they are elected and pressured by the voters. However, since my purpose here is not to change current opinion on corporal punishment, although I care deeply for students, suffice it to say we had a wonderful school where students were taught and disciplined with love and a paddle.

My dear friend, whom I had met when I first began in the school district, was sharing my home. She was a high school counselor and I, a middle school assistant principal. We were inseparable in non-work times. Often when appropriate, we did things together in our work. We knew many of the same people. The school where I worked was a feeder for her school. There were many instances where our paths crossed at work. I had friends, a job I liked, and my life was better than it had ever been.

At age 35 I no longer needed drugs to get through the day. Unfortunately, two years later, that was beginning to change. To prepare and make a speech was something I could do well. To speak with anyone necessary within the scope of my job was not difficult either. However, along the way I missed the skills necessary for light conversation. I was a third wheel when it came to shooting the breeze, and I had a busy social life where I needed to converse with others. To say I was inept is an understatement. I was uncomfortable and afraid others would not like me. I needed a crutch to help me along. I found that a drink or two helped, and with several drinks, I was as comfortable as anyone else in any conversation. No thought was given to my dad's family history of alcoholism. My dad was adamantly against alcohol because he saw what it did with his own father. I was doing just fine, thank you. My drug of choice (it had actually been two years since I had taken pills) changed to alcohol. Fortunately, I only drank in social situations.

Three years after I had become an assistant principal, I became principal of the school. The man who taught me so much retired. It was unusual to become the principal of a school where you were an assistant, but again, much of my life was unusual. I truly loved my new job although there were several other principals who wanted an insider or a male to get the job. Now, someone else had to do the bad stuff as assistant principal, and I got to spoil the kids. Of course, that was not the truth, but I did take some license with them that was not possible as the heavy. I loved working as the teachers' supervisor. I spent many long hours learning new and innovative teaching strategies. I wanted our school to continue being the best, with teachers who were knowledgeable of all teaching methods. It is my opinion that knowledge is not only power; it also creates less stress. Reducing teacher stress became my driving force.

My drive for perfection at work did not change. Year after year I attempted to do a better job than the year before. My fourth year as principal was no different from the first. Now, the teachers might tell you that is not true. They were extremely excited when I was named principal because they already knew me and how I worked. However, they had liked my work with kids; now I began going gangbusters with them! I toned it down as soon as I realized that my zeal was overwhelming, and a new, great relationship began. By this time, my quantity of drinking had greatly increased but continued to be only on social occasions.

Just when my fourth year as principal began, a new superintendent was hired in the district. Wow! I thought I was task oriented. This guy had me beat. Actually, I liked his work ethic, but I was always frightened that I would not live up to his expectations. My sixty plus hour work week grew in hopes of my getting even better. Unfortunately, the new superintendent noticed me too much. Late in the school year, he asked me if I would like to have a job at the administration building. He wanted someone with my work ethic and willingness to do what I believed right, even if it was unpopular. I informed him that I was very happy as a principal and did not desire to make a change.

Employees at my campus knew I had been called to a conference at the administration building, and rumors buzzed that I was going to be moved downtown. I told my faculty that I had been questioned, but that I had said I was very happy where I was. However, when I was summoned two days later, real concern developed both from my faculty and from me. At this meeting, I informed the superintendent that my mother had come to live with me two years before when my dad died. My mother had Alzheimer's disease, and it was difficult enough to meet her needs and be a principal, so it would be impossible at the central office. My roommate was great with my mother and was most helpful. However, I was gone too much as it was, so it would be impossible to change positions. Additionally, I was happy as a principal and believed I could achieve even greater success if left to continue.

After explaining my saga, I went back to my campus and called the teachers together after school. I told them I had informed the superintendent of my situation, and there was nothing to worry about. All was well, I thought. A few days later, I received a letter from the superintendent reassigning me to the central office at the end of the school year (about three weeks later by this time). My heart sank. I went to see the superintendent, and he said he had considered my concerns, but it was his job to run the school district and to place people in the best positions necessary for success of the whole. I was indeed a company person, but I just didn't know how I would juggle my private life.

CENTRAL OFFICE

Four years prior, I had moved within the school district boundary lines when I became a principal. It had been a new prerequisite for my position. Two or three others had encouraged me to fight it since some principals lived outside the district under a grandfather clause. Although there were loopholes that would have been on my side, I was too much of a company person for that. Thus, I moved. My roommate moved with me. When my dad died two years later, my mother came to live with us. She was a delight, but her illness became devastating. We had managed with her living in our home for over two years. It became necessary each day in an effort to keep her safe, to bolt doors with a key, lock windows with an Allen wrench, and switch off the fuses for the stove and oven while we were at work.

After three months at the central office as director of fine arts, I knew something different had to be done. I could not meet my mother's needs and work the hours necessary to attend activities every evening, in addition to my daytime hours. My roommate continued to carry a big load, and our friendship was suffering. That was rightfully so. It was time for a change to be made. The evening before my dad had died, he asked me to promise that I would take care of Mother and never let her go to live with my sister. Therefore, a problem arose when my sister did not want mother to be placed in a nursing home. I saw no reason to tell her about my promise to Daddy. Avoiding family conflict, which was generally true for me, I packed Mother up and moved her to another state fifteen hundred miles away to live with my sister. I had a power of attorney for Mother, but I avoided what I believed would cause great conflict. I felt extreme guilt, but I sent her anyway. It was difficult, but something needed to be done. This was a solution, and I tried to put it out of my mind.

Moving to the central office had not been smooth in ways other than concern for my mother. From the time I was named principal four years earlier, there had been some that resented my appointment. This was a city of just over one hundred thousand people and closely knit for its size. Many others had been there much longer who were believed to have been in line for the position. Additionally, should the first female secondary principal be an implant into the community? That had been four years earlier. Now after only four years, this person had moved to the central office! The acceptance which occurred after my first year as principal, was shattered again.

This new superintendent was making a lot of changes. He did not seem to care how long you had been with the district, who your parents were, or who you knew. Further, he did not seem to care whether he was greatly loved. I might have agreed, considering the changes necessary for my mother, but I saw him as one who truly did what he thought was in the best interest of the school district, whatever the cost. I had never met anyone like him in education, but I had encountered his type in the business world in those who were most successful. (It is not important here, but he wasn't hard to look at either.) It was my opinion that student achievement would improve with the high expectations he held for administrators and teachers. However, everyone did not share my opinion. There was much fear in the district.

Six months after I had been moved to the central office, the superintendent called me into his office and asked me about my lifestyle, since I lived with another woman. I was aware that this had come up after my reassignment downtown. It had been discussed when I was made principal. It had been quiet; no one knew I was aware. I always knew the rumors were there, but I kept it in the back of my mind. As fond of me as my faculty had been when I was promoted to principal after being the assistant, some faculty members sent scouts to find out if I was or if I was not. They had heard the rumors and wanted to know since they knew me best. It happened that one of the female employees and her husband (who taught at the high school across town) were coming to dinner as a thank you for helping us move. They were recruited to be the scouts. They reported back that I was not. I have forgotten now these seventeen or more years later, but someone told me about the plan after its completion, and it was painful to hear. Now, four years later, the superintendent was asking about my lifestyle.

My response was more of a question than an answer. I told him I loved the person with whom I lived very much. We were as true companions as any two people could be. We were inseparable. We loved each other's families and spent time with them as well. We were closer than sisters and most married couples. If those things made me gay, I was, but if it took sex, I was not. I further told him I was just not the marrying kind. My current life was fulfilling.

The superintendent looked at me and said, "That's good enough for me. I'm making you an assistant superintendent for administration. You will be supervisor for all school principals." This was certainly a surprise. I had no idea he was considering this new assignment. He had inherited four assistant superintendents when he came to the district. He would reassign the one over administration. I would take the job in administration and continue with fine arts. As I remember, when I was assigned, there were seventeen elementary schools, six middle schools, two high schools, and two special needs schools.

Here I was, an implant who was to supervise all these principals! I had not run from a challenge for many years, but this was something. After all, I left the forging company because I felt inadequate. What would I do now? It was not that I felt incapable of the job, quite the contrary. The problem was how the principals might perceive me. The challenge was on.

The superintendent called a meeting of all principals and central office employees. He began the meeting and told of the reorganization, including making me the number two in the district. Not only was I to supervise principals, but if central office personnel had a problem when he was not available to contact, they were to call me. Oh dear, was everyone to be against me? More challenge. When the superintendent had finished speaking, he asked me to outline my plan for principals and dismissed central office employees back to their offices.

It was obvious that principals were as surprised as I was. I spoke with them over an hour, giving them my spin on things. I informed them of my honor with the job. Additionally, I had gotten the job because those who had worked for me at my campus had made me look so good that the superintendent thought me responsible. I was spoiled with the reputation my faculty had given me. Further, I completely expected I would continue to be applauded, but now as a result of their performance, not my faculty. Then, I provided some thoughts for the future and asked for input from others.

Actually, everyone was gracious. I'm sure it was not love, but they were gracious nonetheless. After all, I was the one who was responsible for their performance appraisal. As time went by, however, many grew to more than accept me, a few did not. Indeed, I had been hired to be the heavy once more. My business background and task-oriented way of working made me a prime candidate for the job. There were principals who were not working up to the superintendent's expectations, and it was my job to shape them up or ship them out. For the most part, those who needed attention were older principals who had functioned well in a different time under different leadership and expectations. Now, as hard as I tried, three of these principals did not change. The decision was to transfer them to what were considered lesser principalships. I was too much of a company person to tell them I was simply carrying out the superintendent's directions. Some, I am sure, recognized my plight, but others thought I should be unwilling to do those bad things, because they would be incapable of carrying them out if it were their job. It is so difficult for people in the education business to hurt others. For some reason, they do not want to recognize the effect weak teachers have on students. In earlier times, kids managed to get through without apparent harm after having some less-than-dynamic-teachers. Today, however, with the unbelievable expectations, harm comes quickly. At any rate, most principals have not been in the dog-eat-dog business world, but they do recognize the difficult plight of a teacher, so they turn their heads. After all, principals are simply promoted teachers whom we expect to have a heart. Most teachers are good. Many who are not could greatly improve if the time were taken to provide guidance. Many principals are either incapable or unwilling to take the necessary time to help. In all fairness, I must admit the time constraints for principals are tremendous.

All thoughts were not related to work. After I had been in the new job but a short time, mother came to visit for a week at Christmas. She had been out of state three months. When she arrived, she did not look as good physically, but her dementia did not seem as severe. My heart broke, however, when she asked if she could please come home. Not wanting to tell her I just could not take care of her, I told her we would see. I wish so much I could go back and tell her the truth. Why my dad had asked me to promise to keep her here has never been known to me. It is my guess he wanted her to stay in Texas rather than move 1500 miles away. He and mother had lived their lives in Texas and had many friends he would have chosen for her to be near. At any rate, the week with my mother was memorable. I have cherished those memories these fourteen and a half years since. I grieve for having sent her away, but we all have things in our lives we wish we could reverse. I have many!

Five months later, I received a call that my mother had a stroke. It was Wednesday. After attending a school board meeting on Thursday night, I boarded a plane and flew to see my mother. It was in the night when I arrived, but my sister (who had picked me up at the airport) and I went to the hospital to see her. We did not awaken her. The next morning we returned. She was able to walk all over the hospital with me, but the stroke had affected her speaking and swallowing. We stayed with her all day and returned on Saturday morning. After our visit that morning, I decided to get on a plane and return home. Without heroics, she would die. She would not have wanted a feeding tube, so she was released on Monday to return to my sister's house and await death. She died on Wednesday. All those years I feared for this moment; it had now come!

It took a few days for my mother's body to return to Texas for burial. My sister remained with my mother until her body was released for the trip home. In the meantime, my brother and I made arrangements for her funeral. It was a difficult time, but it was a good time to be with my brother. My brother was eighteen when I was born and married when I was three. This was good quality time for me to be with him. My mother was his stepmother; he was nine when our dad married her. The funeral was beautiful. Mother would have approved.

Mother's funeral was on Saturday, a week after my visit with her. On Monday following the funeral, my work continued. We had all gotten through my first couple of years as the assistant superintendent. To say everyone liked me would not be the truth; however, many did respect the sincerity of my work. I grew to truly love principals. It became my desire not only to help them grow, but I worked to hide their flaws from the superintendent the best I could. My work ethic did not change. I was working from 6:30 A.M. until 6:00 P.M., then attending evening activities after dinner (I worked through lunch). I missed one day of work when I flew out of state to see mother, and a half-day to complete her funeral arrangements. Since her funeral was on a Saturday, I did not have to take off work for that. Everyone realized I was dedicated to my job.

Dedicated, but all was not well. My drinking had become very heavy during the third year at the central office. I realized that I was unable to stop. Several attempts had been unsuccessfully made. It was becoming difficult to remember what I needed at work. I constantly made notes to keep up with what I had told whom. I taped conversations so I could review what had taken place. I never drank at work, but I started leaving as soon as I could to get my alcohol fix, get dinner, get sober, and get back to work. It was a vicious cycle. I knew I was in trouble and was trying to figure out how I could get into treatment during a two-week vacation, without anyone knowing what was going on. Denial was not a part of my nature. When I would tell close friends I had a problem, they did not think it was as serious as I did. It is unusual for someone with an alcohol problem to be the one who recognizes a need for help, but I did. In a later chapter, I will provide details about the resolution of the problem. For now, know that I stopped drinking completely during this time without any negative effects. No one ever knew anything except that I refused when offered a drink.

About the time I thought I had a handle on my responsibilities, with life better than it had ever been, the superintendent made a change. He said he wanted me to continue with my current assignment, which included overseeing all campuses and fine arts, and in addition, he was going to add the division of personnel. I would have two divisions, one on each of the two floors of the administration building. There would be a new title. I would be associate superintendent of administration and also of personnel. I cared a great deal for the gentleman who was being reassigned from assistant superintendent for personnel and was disappointed that he was being moved. This was the same person who had interviewed me many years before when I came to the school district. We had a chat, and I realized he did not blame me for the changes. That was a godsend. The greatest problem now was to find time to do the work of three people. I was spending twelve hours a day working as it was.

In order to keep myself on track, I was provided with two offices. We completely redecorated the personnel office. It was beautiful. My secretary was a marvel. Not only did she possess creative ability, she was outstanding as a partner. Principals loved her; she shielded them from me as I shielded them from the superintendent. She could answer questions for me all day long. She came to work early and left late, a divine gift! For her title, she was well paid; for her work and responsibility, she was poorly paid. She stayed in the downstairs office of administration; I started the day downstairs as well. Around ten in the morning, we had coordinated the day and taken care of fires from the previous day. Then, I went up to personnel while she kept the administrative side running. She was also invaluable for the work in personnel, but the work she did with principals was what was of greatest value although there was some overlapping between the two divisions as we ran them. Principals were provided with candidates for job openings from the personnel office. Choices were made at the campus level from those provided. The personnel office screened interviewees and ran background checks on chosen candidates. There were approximately 2,000 employees in the school district. At the time I began as leader of the division, I became the only one who interviewed for teaching positions. There were other employees working for me who interviewed secretarial and custodial positions, but not for those positions which were called professional. That was mine.

My workday began at 6:30 A.M. Around 5:30 or 6:00 P.M. I went home for an hour to eat dinner. I returned to the administration building by 6:30 P.M. and worked until at least 10:00 P.M., which made attending any evening activities at schools impossible. The paper trail necessary in a personnel office is unbelievable. Interviewing is only one time-consuming entity; another is to determine where you will add or remove teaching units, only determined after calculating projections of student enrolments. Every principal wants to add a multitude of teachers to better serve students. There are taxpayers wanting you to spend their money as if it were your own. Conflicts arise. The job is not a simple one.

For me, however, these were happy days. At one point there was a defalcation in the business division and since I had an accounting background, I was asked to coordinate the development of the school district budget for the following year. My part of the coordination lasted about three months. How it was physically accomplished I do not know. I do know that I felt useful and productive. Most principals had decided by this time I was not all bad, and they knew I worked hard to provide them with as much as I could. Certainly, those who were not particularly fond of me would not have told me so; after all, I held their evaluations and salary recommendations in my briefcase. I was aware that many did think I was doing a credible job even if they thought me too task oriented.

After the hiring of a new person for the business division, I was relieved of specific duties for the budget. The new business administrator had like experience in another school district. He was a knowledgeable and easy to get along with person. He was indeed a wonderful addition to the district. I enjoyed the time we spent together as we continued working for district needs. He was invaluable as we worked toward personnel and campus issues. (Again, this was someone who was not hard to look at.)

Several months after having divided my time between the divisions of administration and personnel, we promoted a young man from one of the high school administrative staffs to be director of the personnel department. He was capable and a fast learner. At the end of the following year, he took over the division of personnel, and I had my real job back. At first, I felt like I was missing something. However, soon I was back visiting campuses during the day and attending activities at night. It was necessary to spend a considerable amount of time in the office as well. Paper work is unbelievable. Additionally, I would field thirty or more phone calls each day. That number would have been exponential had my secretary not handled more than I did. Some of these phone calls related to mad mamas. Some were calls from principals warning me they had made a mama mad and what they had done to do so. Some were the mad mamas or dads. When I was unable to help a parent or patron understand our actions, my job was a bummer. Much of the time, however, we came to a meeting of the minds. I tried to realize each time I spoke with an unhappy patron or parent that they were caring people who wanted to make sure their concerns were heard. When I was told it was obvious I cared about kids and for their education, it made that day worthwhile. There were times resolutions were not found. Generally, however, when others recognize that you all want what will be best for not only their child, but for all children, a resolution to the problem can be found to everyone's acceptance, if not satisfaction. Compromises were often made. Whether patron or principal, it seemed to me that I made more concessions than I asked of them, but they sometimes felt just the opposite.

CHANGES, CHANGES

Two more years passed. The superintendent had received a great deal of heat from some school board members for several years. He had made a number of enemies. Not only was he an outsider, he had stirred up a lot of the old timers along the way. When he was hired, every board member was with him one hundred percent. He had warned them at the time he was hired that he was a taskmaster with high expectations. They agreed that many changes needed to be made. They would support him completely. They did. As time went by, however, and school board elections rolled around, folks ran to get rid of the superintendent. First there was one elected, then two, then three. When the fourth came along, it became time for the superintendent to say goodbye. A payoff was necessary because there were still years on his contract. In all, he was there about nine years and for all but the first year, I was with him at the central office. That was quite a long time for a superintendent to stay in one place. I knew enough people in town to understand the reason for the turmoil. Personally, I saw him as someone who truly knew how to run a school district. Untold improvements had taken place; some led to discontentment in the school district. As in any situation, some were happy, some were not. The board over time was not! We (the superintendent and I) differed in our opinions about how you responded to conflict with others. It had been my training to talk things over when there was conflict, or if all else fails, turn and leave, or turn the other cheek. His approach was to enter the conflict full force. That quality, in my opinion, kept him in trouble. It was the downfall of an otherwise brilliant administrator.

In 1994, one year before the superintendent left the district, my long time roommate and I parted after fourteen years. She got married; I got another roommate. My new roomy had three grown and married children. She had been married for thirty-three years to a Baptist minister. She stayed with her husband for many years because of his position but believed that God had finally released her from the marriage. What a talented, knowledgeable lady this was. She had, of course, been very active in church work for years and had not only gained an invaluable knowledge of the Bible; she had a beautiful relationship with the Lord. There was also this wonderful singing voice she used to praise Him.

My friend supported my work endeavors by helping me accomplish something of great importance to me. With my original interest in medicine, for entertainment over thirty years, I read medical books in my meager spare time. For a lay person, I gained greater knowledge than most about symptoms and diseases. My friend was a nursing professor and knew people with whom to speak in order for me to get a new project completed. I wanted selected students to take courses in nursing along with high school courses and graduate with an LVN (licensed vocational nurse) certificate in addition to their diploma. Also, I wanted other groups of students to become certified as an EMT (emergency medical technician). Both programs took a great amount of time to get into place. My friend made many contacts and provided names of those with whom I needed to speak. It was time consuming, and it seemed each call led to another.

We got the program in place after meeting with a state board to bless the project. It was the first of its kind and was placed on probation. The program was to begin the following fall semester with ninth-grade students. These students would be in the program four years for completion. A review would take place at the state level after that time (when the students graduated) to determine whether or not the probation would be removed. The curriculum would be difficult, and students would be unable to get involved in extra-curricular activities because of time constraints. It was further believed that the subject matter was difficult enough that there would be little time for outside activities of any kind. It would take a particular breed of student who would be successful in the program.

After an unbelievable number of hours, the project was complete with students, a certified curriculum, and teachers. It was something of which I was very proud. Whether students could withstand the rigor of the curriculum and the inability to be involved with extra-curricular activities, I did not know. I did think it helpful for students whose parents were unable to send them to college to get a head start on a career. A student completing the LVN program could work while completing an RN certification. A full-time student could be an RN in a year. There are many capable students who end up without jobs and eventually on welfare, who might have made their way if someone had provided the avenue. I wanted our district to provide an avenue. The superintendent supported my efforts as this program was developed. Had there been less turmoil in the district during its inception, I think it would have received greater attention than it did. It may be that I as mother of the program just wanted more.

As time neared for the superintendent to leave, even with uncertainty for the future, I was grateful for the calm that would come.

I did have concern that his departure could change the positive direction in which the district had moved. I had been exposed to many leadership styles in conferences attended over seven or eight years with other superintendents and recognized how few good superintendents there were in the game. It had been different in the business world. The CEO's were for the most part very good leaders with vision for the company. Here we were in education, the most important business, and most of the leaders were weak. From that standpoint, I was grateful for the teaching I had been provided while working with our superintendent. From a personal standpoint, I felt I had been used by the superintendent, but I was also sad that his good qualities were often overlooked. The feeling that he had used me began when he moved me to the administration building at a time devastating for my family. In the business world I have just spoken so highly of, I certainly would have been moved into a new job regardless of my home responsibilities, but I did not expect it in this person friendly vocation. Also, from a career standpoint, it was great. I did think I was trained sufficiently to go anywhere else and be a superintendent if I chose. Additionally, I thought I would be a good one. I was very task oriented, although he had me beat, but my personality was such that I came across differently in some instances than he. In most situations, I was more tolerant. Generally, I worked well with people, considering the parameters of my job. However, I was totally disinterested in going to another district. Having been in the city and school district for over twenty years, it was home. I had no desire to leave the many people I cared for so much.

When the superintendent and the school board prepared for his departure, discussions arose about a replacement. They decided to contract a firm to handle the hiring process and provide them with candidates from which to choose a new superintendent. The board began discussions concerning whom they would place in the superintendent position on an interim basis, as well. It was discussed that some districts hired retired superintendents to fill interim positions when they were to be of short duration. It was thought that filling the position in our district would take a rather long period of time. When asked for my intentions about applying for the position on a permanent basis, I told them I was not interested in applying for the long term. I said I would be willing to serve as superintendent while they looked for another and would continue with my present job (I was used to that). They decided if I was not interested in the position on a permanent basis, that would be the thing to do. They voted to provide me with a small stipend, and off we went. Again, I was used, but I set myself up this time.

As time went by in the position of superintendent, I found that the job was not what I had expected. I was the happiest I had ever been in my entire life. I was at home with the people I loved. To say I loved my job is an understatement. It was even more demanding than when I had been working on the budget, handling both the divisions of administration and personnel, and coordinating fine arts. The time spent speaking with school board members, community leaders, and the myriad of people you do not even know exist, make minutes meld into hours. There were truly not enough hours in the day. What a joy! Those eight months passed faster than most weeks had in my early life and were the best I had lived or thought possible to live.

The school board was wonderful to work with. They were supportive and allowed me to make changes and move on in any way I desired. New programs were added. New committees were developed to enhance the educational process for kids. Teachers were involved in decision making as never before. Parents were included in decision making as never before. Minority groups were providing input as never before. Some central office job descriptions were changed to facilitate coordination with campuses.

With encouragement from community members, parents, teachers, and other administrators, I believed I was the right person for the job. There had been a person who applied for the position whom I believed would be good to work with and for, but the board had not been interested in him. So, looking at how well most current employees worked together (and I had seen who the other possibilities for candidates were) I informed the board that I wanted the job after all.

It was what some school board members wanted to hear; others said they were concerned with what the community would think after they had hired a firm (at a very large price tag) to generate applicants for the position. It was my opinion at the time that it was best for the district, as well as for me, that I remain in the superintendent position. What should the money matter if everyone were better served? Although my desires were not known by a great number of people, it was known by a sufficient number to create the taking of sides. I realized it could turn into a problem if too many knew, and I therefore backed off, not wanting to harm the district in any way. It appeared obvious to me that I should remain as superintendent; however, if the entire board was not on the same page, it would not be best. I decided to accept whomever they chose and do all I could to make that person successful.

When the board had selected a new superintendent, I took him from campus to campus for meetings with each faculty and administration during his first few days. I told them how excited we all were for him to be there and what a wonderful addition he would be for the district. During the first few days, I grew to genuinely like the new guy and thought he might be a healer for the district. As time went by, however, I realized he would basically destroy all the hard work that had been accomplished by prior boards, administrators, and teachers. Unfortunately, it took time for the school board to recognize his weaknesses. He was such a likeable person with all the right things to say about running a district, but it took months for some board members who had handpicked him to be willing to recognize the need to go through the find-a-superinten-dent process again.

It took two years before recognizing he would be better suited for another district, and three years before it was accomplished. During that third year, several board members spoke with me about my turn. It was my opinion that my turn had passed. So much had changed.

RETIREMENT

The state legislature changed retirement rules that year. Over the Christmas holidays, I had read the book *Your Money or Your Life*. As I looked at each graph, and filled out each scenario, I found I could afford to retire. It would be quite a leap for me. I had certainly worked hard, but I felt I could play hard, too! Most said I would be truly miserable in retirement. They thought I would be lost without something to do. Feeling there was nothing to work for anymore, I decided it was time to hang it up and did so.

At fifty-four years old, everyone thinks you should be gainfully employed. I was not interested. However, it took me most of the first year after retirement to adjust to feeling not needed. It had taken me many years to think myself useful; now I had to decide what to do. I had lost my love; there was nothing I wanted to do. I had never been much of a traveler. Also, I had an aging dog whom I dearly loved. After a trip to Disney World for ten days, three months after retirement, I left him for no more than two nights at a time. Even when he was young he had separation anxiety; now that he was old, he became so ill I hardly left him at all.

After the first year passed, I wondered why I had ever pined for my prior work. In fact, I felt like so many retirees who say they wonder how they ever found time to work. Anita (my roommate) and I filled our days with fun. Through much of my life, I said I wanted to be a bum with a paycheck. That had come true! We had moved to live on the lake in a small, quaint town. We were active in church and could be as social or nonsocial as we desired. Oh, what most people would give to have our blessings. As one thing or another arose that was a problem for us, most would have said we were picking at nits.

During the third year of retirement, we were asked to become more deeply involved in our church work. We sang in the choir, and my roommate was high on everyone's list to teach Sunday school classes. We had served on committees and been involved to a great extent, but now we had been asked to serve in more official capacities. I was asked to be financial secretary for the church, Anita to be a deacon. We were both honored for the requests to serve.

Two couples in the church went to the pastor and suggested the position of deacon be reconsidered. It was acceptable to be responsible for the church stewardship fund, but the Bible noted that a deacon was to be someone who had not been divorced. Further, they were considering someone who lived with another woman!

When we became aware of the couples' concerns, we both declined our positions. It was acceptable to these couples for Anita to teach Sunday school classes and me to handle the financial responsibilities but not to serve as a deacon. This did (and does) not compute with me. A teacher touches and molds thoughts and lives far more than a deacon. We were very quiet about our feelings, but unfortunately, the elders and other church leaders continued to encourage us not to pay any attention to the few who had voiced objections. However, since the last thing we wanted to do was create problems, we decided to return to a church we attended earlier in another city. It was a long drive, but there had not been a problem with us in that congregation, and it was a wonderful place to worship.

Satan used our leaving the church to create more problems than while we were there. Humanness is indeed a stumbling block for God's work! More about this time in my life will be detailed in a later chapter. Suffice it to say that the continued calls from elders and other church leaders were appreciated. Were I able to go back and try the other route and not leave, I would. Running from a problem is not my style, but it seemed best for the church at the time, and that was our desire.

A little over a year after leaving the church, I began what was to be many visits with physicians. That was in 2001, as detailed earlier, concerning how I came to know I had a tumor. Church members and leaders had continued, since our leaving the church, to call and tell us there was a gap without our being there. We had always thanked them and moved on. However, after finding that the tumor was malignant, I called the pastor who had recently retired. I told him of the cancer and short life expectancy. I wanted him to conduct the funeral if and when I died. I wanted to be on his and the church's prayer list. Immediately, calls came by the multitude. The interim pastor made several phone calls and visits. After I became well enough to attend, we began going back to our church.

At this writing, it has been a year and a month since my surgery. It has been interesting to observe behaviors of many who have watched my healing miracle. Two or three months after returning to church, I was feeling so well, someone asked me if I was sure I had not been misdiagnosed. (Anita had prophesied this would probably happen; it did!) I responded with the credentials of the three well-known and highly respected cancer centers located throughout the United States having confirmed the diagnosis. We always think every miracle is a coincidence, a fluke, or a mistake. Surely, God must grieve for our lack of belief.

JESUS IN MY LIFE

Reflecting on my past has been both happy and sad for me. To this point, I have provided the facts from my birth to the present time. Now, I want to fill in the gaps that I believe are the result of a living God.

As mentioned earlier, my parents were very devout Southern Baptists. Whenever the church doors were open, we were there. It did not make me happy to be pulled from my outside activities on Sunday evening to return to church; I had enough church during the morning. But, shy as I was and as much trouble as I was for everyone at school less than a year later, I wanted to accept Jesus around the time of my sixth birthday. My parents were concerned that I knew not what I was doing because of my young age, and asked the pastor to speak with me. After speaking with me, he told them he thought my profession of faith and baptism would be appropriate. I was shy and deathly afraid of water, so I did not want the baptism part. After being convinced it was required, I submitted. I remember to this day, however, how truly petrified I was the night of my baptism. I did go through with it and felt the greatest sense of relief after it was over. I did it for Jesus, I got it, and that was that.

Looking back and thinking about my childhood years and my totally unacceptable behavior, I realize how I completely separated my actions from my belief in Jesus. Jesus loved me just as I was. No matter how much I was told that Jesus was not pleased that I did this or that, I thought what I heard at church was correct, not what I was told at home. At church, I was very shy but I did pay attention. Since I would not speak out or answer questions, even though I often knew answers, I was afraid I might be wrong and considered myself stupid. Remembering how I thought and felt was invaluable in the work I eventually would pursue.

Through the elementary school years, my behavior at church was good, although I was quiet. I loved Jesus and believed He was my Savior. As mentioned, what I did at school was a completely different matter. I did not see what difference it made to God whether or not I did my work, and I did not think one way or another about what He thought of my bad decisions. Also, it appeared to me that Sunday morning church should be all that was necessary. What I thought did not matter, of course, and it seemed to me we were always at church. Except for the actual church services, I was most uncomfortable with Sunday school, training union, and girl's auxiliary. You had to answer questions or get up in front of the group to do something. That was not for me. For the most part, the leaders allowed me be a non-entity. That was better than participating, but I still felt uncomfortable.

By the time junior high came along, I would sneak off from church on Thursday nights and go to the city recreation center. Yes, this Baptist learned to dance. I went to the center for over a year and was never caught. This was church visitation night, and you were either in visitation teams, or you attended study sessions. When I look back, I realize that someone had to know I was not in attendance. They must have taken pity on me and not told my parents. There were some kids whose parents allowed them to fool around on the church grounds until time to go home. My session leaders probably thought I was with other kids. To have stayed outside with other kids who were not in organized sessions would have been totally unacceptable, to go to the recreation center would have been beyond thought. There is definitely <u>no way</u> my parents knew.

Each summer when it was time for church camp, my parents tried to get me interested in going. I did attend one or two hayrides along the way because I truly liked the youth director. He was really good with this shy misfit. The last year I was eligible to go with a particular age group to church camp, I decided to go. For several years the youth director had encouraged me to go and told me it would not be like school or even Sunday school, but I had not wanted to go. Now, however, I decided to give it a try. I remain convinced it was a miracle that I went when I did. My parents were delighted. The bus trip was fun. We sang along the way, and after we got there, the camp chaperone with whom I was assigned was someone I felt comfortable with. On the first day, I met a boy and fell in love. Boys were always easy for me to talk with. Unlike at school, at camp you ate with a boy if you liked, as well as were with him at other times. At school, boys walked you to class, but boys ate with boys and girls ate with girls. That always made lunch difficult for me. I had a boyfriend at school, but I was alone at lunch. The following year, only a short time later, I think it may have been as a result of church camp, the girls from church decided to invite me to sit with them. At any rate, I spent all my camp time with my new boyfriend. I had a boyfriend at home, but this was really fun. He was from another city, so no one had to know!

Church camp was truly a wonderful experience for me. I actually blossomed forth on several occasions during that week; unfortunately however, when I returned home, I was back to my old self as far as my shyness was concerned. It had been easy to speak with others at church camp. Also, one day at the end of the morning services, we were asked to raise our hands if we would like to be a part of the evening service and be hypnotized. I actually held up my hand. Looking back, it was a miracle that I even held up my hand. For some reason, it was not threatening to me. I was chosen as one of ten! This, too, was a miracle since there were probably five hundred or more there and many wanted to be hypnotized. At any rate, I was hypnotized. We were instructed to do several things under hypnosis, and it was fun. I remember us being told to think of the funniest thing we had ever heard. I laughed uncontrollably no matter how hard I tried not to. It was certainly positive and has been a wonderful memory in my life.

After returning home from camp, even though I remained shy and stupid, I was a new person. I was getting ready to enter the ninth grade, and my life had made a definite turn for the better during the past year. Now I had come home from church camp with a new drive for life. The girls from church had been really kind to me and invited me to do several things with them during camp. I spent most of my time with my guy, but it was nice to be asked. In addition, I had moved to a new depth with the Lord. I felt some kind of call for something. I did not know of anything a Baptist girl could do except be a foreign missionary. I could not talk, I was not very smart, and I had a cigarette habit I thought might be impossible to kick. However, this spurred my first attempt to quit.

My prayer life deepened to the point that I talked with God off and on all the time, the first two or three weeks after returning home from camp. I would lie on my bed at night looking out the window at the moon and stars while engaging in conversation with God. I was in love with Him. As has always been true with me, I had too many complications to be as high on the mountain top as was warranted. It was impossible to get the feeling there was something I was supposed to do off my mind.

One night after I had gone to bed, I looked out the window (I had my bed beside the window and my head in it) and saw a beautiful full moon. It was an awe-inspiring time for me. As I talked with the Lord, I told Him it would really be difficult for me to be a missionary. First of all, I could not talk. Secondly, I was not smart enough. Thirdly, I was a smoker. I had managed to stop smoking for a week or two, but it seemed impossible to stop. During my conversation with God, I spoke about my continuing to feel that He was calling me to do something. I needed a sign. In times past, I had "fleeced" (in Sunday school I had learned about Bible characters who fleeced by asking God to show a sign) God and sometimes there had been an answer. I told Him that night that I really needed to hear from Him. I continued with the thought that the only possible thing He might be calling me to do would be mission work. Soooooo, I asked Him to let me see a flash of lightning in the sky by the time I counted to ten if He were calling me to the mission field. I began to count one, two, three, and so on very slowly until I reached nine. Then I slowed down to a stop to give Him plenty of time before I said ten. After a very long pause, I said ten. Then, I gave God more time after I said ten in case He was still thinking about it. Nothing happened. I continued to talk and told Him I needed to know He was there. Something really special was going on in my life, and I needed an answer.

At an earlier time when I was younger, on at least two or three occasions and perhaps more, I had prayed to the Lord fervently to restore my mother's hearing. I would ask and then go to sleep knowing that the following morning I would wake up and my mother would be able to hear. I was extremely disappointed the first time I asked and the following morning there had been no change. I decided my faith must not be strong enough. The second time I asked, I was completely positive that it would be restored this time. Again, there was no hearing. I did not lose faith; I just thought there was something wrong with the way I must be making my request. Eventually, I decided it was not God's will because I knew He could do it if He wanted to.

Now, I was asking God for a sign. I do not remember my exact feelings these forty or so years ago, but I do remember how desperately I needed a sign from God. I remember well how I asked that He let me know He was there, and I continued to count to fifteen. When I reached the number fifteen, there were fireworks blazing across the sky. I had asked for a flash; I got a spectacular event. Wow! He was there! This was on a night without a cloud in the sky.

I slept very little that night wondering if I should tell anyone about the lightning, and feeling great excitement. I did not suspect anyone would believe me, and again, my memory is clouded concerning the next morning except that I did tell my mother. She believed me. In fact, as I recollect, there was an article in the newspaper the following day about some unusual happening in the sky the previous night. My credibility had done a complete turnaround since my trip to church camp, and I was believed even before the newspaper arrived that evening. I did not tell anyone else, and except for my retelling of this event as an adult on several occasions, to the best of my recollection, it was not mentioned at home. It is sad that such true miracles are not discussed for fear your credibility will be questioned. I wonder about God's sadness that we did not scream it from the rooftops!

As often happens, soon my normal life took its toll on my miracle, and it was only a memory. It was a good thing, however, that my somewhat wild lifestyle had been so beautifully interrupted with camp and a real-God encounter. I continued to live a somewhat double life. Now, not only did I go to church as I always had, I began to read more and more from the Bible. Also, an evangelist held a revival at our church soon after camp (the actual time frame has been forgotten), and I was most impressed. I listened to every word. He was rather young, handsome, and was not from the usual mold of our church. We were a large all white (usual in those days) congregation, and this young man was Mexican (today we would say Hispanic, but I remember he called himself a Mexican). Later, his brother who was also an evangelist led a revival. I was enthralled with both. My parents bought copies of their sermons at my bidding. When I was the only one at home, I would preach these sermons to the knots on the knotty pine walls in our living room. After awhile, I developed my own sermons. My sermons were not well planned; they were impromptu. I always used Scripture, but I do not remember if the Scriptures were determined at random, or if I used those I knew well.

My split existence continued for a short time. Soon, my wilder friends were dismissed, and I spent most of my time with my church friends. I considered the most sinful thing in my life to be my cigarette habit (my church friends remained unaware). I tried a time or two to stop, but it was hard, and my boyfriend being a smoker made it doubly hard. He attempted to stop as well, but he didn't make it either. He was nine years older than I, had already been in the army, and had a job in the big world. On second thought, some might say my wild driving was worse than my smoking because many were at risk when I was behind the wheel.

When I was sixteen or seventeen years old, a significant event occurred while driving the car. I always knew there was something unusual about this event, but I had reached an acceptable explanation that seemed to satisfy me in the absence of a better one. My sister had married and moved to the northeast, but on this particular occasion, she was visiting. It was during the summer, and I was keeping the car hot. One evening, my sister, my best girlfriend from church, and I were joyriding. There was a really large dip in front of my high school. We often got up to speeds of 95 to 100 MPH before reaching the crest of the hill at the top of the dip. On this particular evening, I looked down at the speedometer and it read 95. We were nearing the crest of the hill, and we all saw a white Volkswagen backing out of a driveway approximately 100 to 150 feet from our position. The worst place a driver could go is to the floorboard, but that is where I went. My two passengers, one in the back seat, one on the other side in the front, placed themselves in a duck-and-cover position with their heads between their knees and hands over their heads. We were all preparing for the crash. It did not come. Almost simultaneously, the four hubcaps popped off the car. The car had stopped. The three of us got out and looked for the Volkswagen. It was nowhere in sight: it had vanished! Two of the hubcaps were rolling toward the curb and we retrieved them as well as the other two that lay near the car. We were unable to get them back on. I remember telling my dad that they just popped off. He did not buy it, but my sister supported my story.

Through the years, I accepted the fact that it was a mystery where the Volkswagen had gone. The only explanation I could conjure up for the hubcaps popping off was that the car had moved at such a high rate of speed between the Volkswagen and a very large tree in the yard across but next to the street, that the suction created the action. To the reader, this sounds as stupid as I thought I was as a kid, but when something unexplainable occurs, we can come up with a lot of things. For these past forty years, I have told the story many times with wonder. I knew there was a miracle; I just could not piece together what it was. Only in this past year has the Lord revealed to me what really happened. It is interesting as well, that I remember some things now that I had not thought about over these many years. I did not think about them because it would make the story even more unbelievable. I now remember that when I climbed back into the driver's seat, the car was sitting even with the driveway where the car had pulled out, only a few feet farther down the road than the tree. By the time I reached the floorboard, the car would have been near or past the point where impact should have occurred, with the vehicle moving only a little more slowly than the 95 I had seen. The car could not have possibly stopped for a very long distance nor would it have stayed in a narrow street. It would most likely have run off the road into a house, that is if you discount hitting the car. Where did the car go? How had our car stopped immediately when it was going 95 miles per hour?

Over the past six months, two books about angels have been placed in my path. I have never thought a lot about angels. The Bible says angels are real, so I believe in them. I believe in Michael and Gabriel for sure. But in these books I read, there was story after story from reasonable people who believed in angels. Billy Graham wrote the first book I read. I probably would not have read anything about angels by anyone else at first, because I did not think much about their presence with us today. I am often skeptical about things I do not understand. I have not seen a winged humanlike creature to this day.

Now, I do believe in angels! Both books detail incidents that are impossible to understand as being devoid of miraculous happenings; it must be that angels are alive and well! None of the angels I read about had wings either, but many were seen. I did not see the angels who must have held our car in the air, suspended above the Volkswagen, long enough for it to get out of sight, then drop our car to the street just hard enough for all four hubcaps to pop off almost simultaneously. This is my new explanation, and I think it a lot more accurate than the first. It would be hard to express my current appreciation for miracles, angels, and belief that God must really grieve that we explain away all the many things He personally takes care of for us. I explained it away for forty years. Only when I recently asked my sister for her assessment of what happened (we had not mentioned it over these forty plus years) that I understood what had truly taken place. She said she remembered well that we had flown over the car because she felt the car hit the ground, and the hubcaps popped off. Knowing that I had driven over the dip at over 100 miles per hour and the wheels did not come off the ground, our flying over the car had never been a part of my assessment of the situation. She had to make sense of something that made no sense in context for her mind. I had done the same. Now, with both versions and a little help from the Lord, I am amazed to realize that we, too, have an angel story.

SERIOUSLY ILL

A year or so after the car incident, when I was in the twelfth grade, I began experiencing health problems. My parents took me to doctors and a plethora of tests were ordered. The diagnosis was leukemia. Several blood specialists saw me, and each offered the same assessment. After a short time, I became considerably worse. I was taking gigantic quantities of steroids and they did not agree with my system. It was determined that the steroids should be discontinued because I would only live a short time, probably about three months.

The diagnosis was later changed when it appeared I was not going to die. It is not my intention here to reiterate this illness since it was detailed earlier. I bring it up again to mention that a devastating illness disappeared. Was it truly misdiagnosed? Was it a miracle? At the time, it would have been difficult to believe it anything other than a misdiagnosis. Today, however, with the preponderance of happenings in my life, I cannot put a miracle aside. We often think miracles probably don't happen at all, but certainly they do not happen to us!

It would not be fair to leave out the part I believe prayer played in my healing. As mentioned earlier, we attended a very large church. Every Wednesday evening, our church held a prayer meeting. At this service, the pastor gave a short sermon preceded by a list of those who needed prayer. For some time, my name had been on the prayer list, and all in attendance prayed for me. Those who chose to wrote a note on a postcard, turned it in, then the postcards were mailed out from the church. I received many, many postcards from church members who were praying for me.

This was again true when my spleen was removed during the third year of work on my bachelor's degree. I will discuss this surgery now with the illness that preceded it even though it occurred somewhat later. It continues to point to the power of prayer. The Good Book says in James 5:16b of the King James Version "the effectual fervent prayer of a righteous man availeth much." In the New Living Translation, James 5:16 reads "Confess your sins to each other and pray for each other so that you may be healed. The earnest prayer of a righteous person has great power and wonderful results." I believe a lot of righteous folks were praying for me, and it availed healing.

As noted, my spleenectomy is not in chronological order, but I mention it here because prayer from the same church was lifted up for me each week during this time, probably about three years after onset of the original illness.

When I went to the hospital to have my spleenectomy performed, I felt well for the most part. My platelet count, although low, was much improved. I had previously been through an appendectomy and tonsillectomy, and both were a breeze. Hospitals were old hat to me, and this would be no different.

During surgery, however, there was a serious problem. My spleen was nicked without the surgeon being aware. By the time he recognized the severe blood loss, my heart had stopped, as had my breathing. There was no blood available in the operating room, and it took awhile to get it there. In the meantime, they performed open heart massage in an attempt to keep my heart beating. I do not understand all the ins and outs that came after. I only know the surgeon told my parents they had a difficult time because there was little blood to circulate with CPR. I had been without sufficient oxygenation for a period considerably greater than five minutes. The exact amount of time it took to get blood to the OR is not remembered now, but I do know he was concerned about the possibility of brain damage. Wow, it is a good thing I was asleep! I had just gotten over thinking I was genetically brain damaged! When the surgery was completed, heart rate and breathing restored, a period of waiting took place where neither the surgeon nor my parents knew whether or not I really would be brain damaged.

Many people report they have out of body experiences, or see white lights in a tunnel when near death. I have always said I did not experience anything like that. I did not, although I do remember having some sort of belief that I was either dead or dying. I was experiencing extreme peace. I had a body; I think my own. I only am aware that when I did eventually wake up after the surgery (it was a long period of time), I was extremely disappointed that I was still alive. This was during one of the better times in my life. I had not completely given up the thought of working in the field of medicine, I had confidence that I could succeed, and I had friends to enjoy. But something had happened while I was out that was even better. I do not remember what my experience was, only that I liked the thought of dying.

Again, it is my belief that prayer was the answer, not only to my living through the surgery but also the lack of brain damage. A series of tests were performed to confirm my mental ability. This gave me new proof of my ability. Although I will speak much more about being chosen and set apart for God as *the* reason I believe all the miracles have happened in my life, I believe prayer played a mighty role in these episodes as well.

Chapter 14

MORE MIRACLES

In an effort to discuss my blood problem within the same chapter, I jumped ahead to discuss the spleenectomy. I will now digress back to the beginning of college and the chronology of miracles in my life.

The first year after high school I did not attend college. I began college in the summer following the year I worked for an insurance company. Continuing college courses in the fall, I met a man who had a profound effect on my life. I do not now believe it was coincidence for all classes I needed to be full that semester. Never in the remainder of my college work (which all totaled after this point was well over 200 credit hours) did I encounter a conflict of this magnitude. Here I was, a freshman with a class conflict! I have thought it unusual these many years although I never considered how truly unusual it was until recently. It was a necessity to have me meet this professor. He influenced my life to a greater extent than perhaps any human being before or since. It has seemed that the right person has always come along, but this timing proved to be a pivotal point for so many things that happened from then until now.

My relationship with this teacher was ongoing for many years. The Lord used him in a mighty way in my life. The profound effect he had on me revolved around my shyness and feeling of stupidity. Without the changes that occurred over the following four years, my life would have been completely different. I may well have remained a shy misfit who would have eventually committed suicide—I will never know. I will mention here that I had contemplated suicide several times in earlier years. For the purposes of this book, that topic will not be revived. My life took such a different turn that suicide does not seem to have a place as I look back.

During the time I took speech and drama classes in college, skills consistently developed. When I was well prepared, my fear of inadequacy and inability were on the back burner. Where there had earlier been zero confidence, it had blossomed. There is no way I will ever again believe all these events were a result of coincidence or happenstance. The hand of the Lord is written all over it! I had always realized this was a pivotal part of my life, and without it I would have spent my life lacking the ability to converse about anything other than on a superficial level at best. I wonder if I had become a surgeon whether or not I would have had adequate confidence in my relationships with my patients to show empathy. I have encountered more than one surgeon who was all business and have wondered if I would have been the same.

Therein lies what I believe to be another miracle. With the pace I have kept during these past thirty-five years, I could have easily withstood the rigors of medicine, but it was not to have been, and I am *so* glad! In public school administration a la Sharon, the hours were twenty-four each day. The few I spent in bed were not sleeping: they were in preparation for the following day. Sleeping has never been my "long suit." I thank God for providing me with the memories I have of working with parents and teachers in the pursuit of educated, well-behaved children. It has been far more fulfilling than medicine might have been. Without my miracle professor,

I also do not know what I would have done when I was told it would not be possible for me to continue my pursuit of medicine. I do not believe I would have considered education without him or some other angel in my path. The stage had been set. The timing was right.

An educator is what I was meant to be. It is like there was something hovering above my head throughout life that kept me moving in a particular direction. I kept veering off the path, but that hand appears to have returned me back to the chosen way when I strayed too far. Even the do not rehire in my file in one of the school districts was perhaps a miracle (I will come back to that later).

There were times those straying paths were for a purpose, unknown to me at the time. One of those times was in California. When I lived in California, my depression was at a high. Life had no meaning. All I wanted was to come home. Today, I realize my life in California was for a very important reason. For the past thirty plus years, I have been deeply interested in Bible prophesy.

While we were in California, we joined a small fundamentalist Baptist church. I had neither attended a small nor fundamentalist church before. There were fewer than a hundred people in attendance on Sunday mornings. At the time we joined, I really did not think about the difference between Southern Baptists and other Baptists. Soon, and *very* soon, I recognized that it was by far stricter than my experiences throughout life in the Southern Baptist church. Here, it was not acceptable to even go to the beach or wear a swimsuit, but that was all right with me. I liked this church, its people, and I would attempt to live within the guidelines of their beliefs. I was extremely depressed anyway, so what was another no? Because I was alone most hours of the day, six days a week, I went to every activity the church offered.

One Sunday morning, we had a guest preacher who spoke on the Second Coming of Christ. I was in the habit of taking notes during the sermon, but notes were particularly important this day. We went from Revelation to Isaiah, from Isaiah to Daniel, from Daniel to one of the four gospels, from the gospels back to Revelation. Movement among these books went from one to another. I wrote down Scriptures as fast as I could. There was little time to read and understand what was in each passage. I tried at first but decided to write down all the Scriptures and dig through them at home.

What a sermon this was! So often in those days when sermons were preached on the book of Revelation, a picture of gloom and doom was presented. It was scary stuff to think about. Wars, pestilence, misery, and death were not happy things. At least that was the general impression of the time. This sermon, however, was not at all gloom and doom. It highlighted the fact that these things had to happen in order for Christ to return. At Christ's return, all would be well! Wellness should be our goal, only to be reached when our Lord came back to earth.

The rapture of the church was talked about. Although the word rapture is not in the Bible, the catching away is. The word rapture comes from Latin and means to be caught up. I like Hal Lindsey's calling it the great snatch. I had not heard of Hal Lindsey when I was in California, but his name is a household word in my house now. At the time, I had heard of some distant notion of Jesus coming and taking us to be with Him, but a true picture of the catching away was not a part of my repertoire of knowledge. Whatever it was, it was far off, and we were not to think about it much anyway. According to Matthew 24:36, "no one knows the day or the hour when these things will happen." Matthew 24:37–39 states, "When the Son of Man returns, it will be like it was in Noah's day. In those days before the flood, the people were enjoying banquets and parties and weddings right up to the time Noah entered his boat. People didn't realize what was going to happen until the Flood came and swept them all away. That is the way it will be when the Son of

Man comes." In Revelation 16:15 it says, "Take note: I will come as unexpectedly as a thief! Blessed are all who are watching for me, who keep their robes ready so they will not need to walk naked and ashamed." Sometimes we do not mention, however, that in Luke 12:37–38 Jesus says, "There will be special favor for those who are ready and waiting for his return. I tell you, he himself will seat them, put on an apron, and serve them as they sit and eat! He may come in the middle of the night or just before dawn. But whenever he comes, there will be special favor for his servants who are ready." In the first half of Matthew chapter 24, Jesus foretells many things to happen just before he comes again. Then, in Matthew 24:32–33 He says, "Now learn a lesson from the fig tree. When its buds become tender and its leaves begin to sprout, you know without being told that summer is near. Just so, when you see the events I've described beginning to happen, you can know his return is very near, right at the door."

Some of the statements are considered to refer to the Second Coming and others to the catching away. I am certainly not, nor do I pretend to be, a theologian. I simply am one who has a deep love for Bible prophesy. It was born in California. It is my belief that the sermon on prophesy was the purpose for my living in California. I have only come to this conclusion during the past year while reflecting prayerfully on my life. Before this time, I could find no reason for the time I spent in California. Perhaps there were other benefits as well; I simply am grateful to have thought of one. In my life, it has been a big one. Only God knows whether or not the Lord will come again in a time frame considered soon by the population. I believe He will. Whether or not I am correct is really not important. What is important is that I believe my interest in prophesy over these thirty-one years has been purposeful for my life. It was more than a minor miracle that I heard the sermon. I have neither heard one before nor one like it since. I would have missed out on so many blessings as well as the hundreds of hours I have spent reading about Bible prophesy. I think it also important to believe the Lord's timing is always correct and that His return will be at a perfect time as well. Some do not believe He is coming back at all. At one time in my life, that would have destroyed the entire foundation of all I believed about Christianity. However, I have come to believe that were there nothing beyond this life, my life has indeed greatly benefited from the relationship I have with the Lord. I do, however, hope to and *believe I will* see Him face to face.

Getting to return home from California was a mountain top experience. We returned from California with $88, the relatively new Cadillac we had when we went, our clothes, and hope for the future. God was good, and it was only eight or nine months after returning that we were able to buy a house. The house was even nicer than the one we had sold to move west, probably worth $150,000 on the North-Central Texas market today. It is somewhat unusual that we were able to buy this house in such a short time. I did not think about it then, but I realize it was a gift from God. Also, when we needed for me to get a job to buy equipment, I was hired in a good paying management job where I was the first female ever hired directly into management. I had no management experience, so how did this happen? All of these many things have come to my mind during this past six months. Looking at individual events as they happened was one thing—when viewed in totality, quite another. Never before have I looked at my past with such scrutiny. So many things just do not add up. Something made these things happen. I would not have been capable of steering this path. They all worked together, however and moved me in a specific direction.

After about two years, I quit my management job to work once more in the silk-screen business. It was basically a two person operation. (My husband did the work of two or three, but I count him only as one. He is a very talented person.) As recounted in an earlier chapter, soon after quitting my management job, I decided to file for divorce. I therefore needed to find a new job.

Amazingly enough, I applied for a bookkeeping position which quickly turned into a really good job. After five months, as detailed earlier, I remarried my husband, believing that I had made a horrible mistake by divorcing. It was not long before I again believed marriage was a mistake, but I decided to grin and bear it.

As I look back, two management jobs fell in my lap. Again, I had never looked at how unlikely that was. Management was a natural for me, but I was educated to be a teacher. God's timing dictated that I once again look in the direction of teaching. The desire to teach came when we materially had almost everything we wanted. I also became uncomfortable with all the responsibility in the accounting position. I believed a CPA would be a better choice for that position. I find this timing interesting as well. Why had I held that job for two years growing in material wealth, then deciding all of a sudden that I was not qualified for the job?

A miracle occurred when I began looking for a teaching position. First of all, I thought it unusual at the time that I had gone to two or three school districts without getting a job. I only got an interview in one district and was given inaccurate information about hiring practices.

As noted in an earlier chapter, when I called a principal in the school district where I taught five years before, I found there was a do not rehire in my file. This information had obviously been passed on to districts where I sent an application. I used the previous personnel office as a reference, believing my record to be sound. Although I experienced unbelievable anxiety during this time, I realize now it was for a purpose.

Today, I find it interesting that the personnel director of the district where I was hired to teach just happened to be in the outer office when I picked up an application one particular day during my lunchtime. It was probably because I was able to speak with him personally and explain my do not rehire, as well as previous applications, that he considered hiring me. That had to have come from a higher power. The personnel director must have taken pity on me and decided to give me a chance. That too is most unusual. It is difficult to fire educators. Extensive documentation is necessary to remove a poor teacher. Hiring someone with a "do not rehire" just does not happen! Perfect timing—I met an angel. More coincidence? At some point, even coincidence gets us to scratch our heads. It was *my* life I am talking about here, and until this year when the Lord unfolded all these memories in sequence, I was as blind to most events being miracles as some readers may be after reading my account. I recognized this particular event as a miracle when it occurred, but most miracles I did not see. Even though I recognized it as a miracle, I simply thanked the Lord that He had been so good to me. Each memory I put on paper now makes me shake my head in shame. Oh, how we grieve the Lord through our ignorance and unbelief! It appears to me now that my whole life has been miracle after miracle.

Although I recognized my being rehired in teaching was a miracle, I did not know the extent. I simply thought it a miracle that anyone took a chance after the note in my previous file. Not only was it beyond belief that I was hired at all, but I was hired in a fast-growing district where numerous schools would be built in a very few years. My business background was appreciated, and the skills I had learned were noticed. After the many experiences gained in the five years I was away from teaching and the maturity that went along with time, I was good at just about anything I tackled, and I knew it. The kids in my classes learned and enjoyed my approach. Other teachers were sometimes jealous because the kids liked me, but they were professional about it.

Actually, at this time I was pushing myself on a personal level with other teachers. I was shy and felt quite inept in light conversation. Many thought me cold until they knew me. That was not true for my students; they knew me well and knew I liked them. I had no qualms telling students anything they wanted to know about me. Many teachers are hesitant to let kids know them too well because kids often take advantage through manipulation and presenting get-away-with behavior. That was not a problem for me. Even that gives pause for wonder. Perhaps I'm the only teacher I have ever known just like me. I was a strict disciplinarian who got close to students. Where did this most unusual trait come from, I wonder?

Two years after I began teaching again I was encouraged to move into administration. I was a woman, and at that time it was very unusual for a woman to pursue a career in administration other than elementary school. At first I was too enamored with the kids in my classroom to be interested, but with continued encouragement, decided to make the change. Had I been in any other school district, it is unlikely that these changes and the encouragement that went along with them would have taken place.

When I was hired as an assistant principal, even the school to which I was assigned laid a foundation for my future. Had I been assigned with my principal who encouraged me to make the change in the first place, the one who asked for me to be assigned as his assistant, the outcome would have been far different. It is most unusual that I was assigned to someone who did not ask for me, but it happened. It had to happen this way for me to become the principal after three years. At that time, it was almost unheard of to become a principal after only three years' experience in administration. I certainly was not the first, but it was very unusual to say the least. I was a woman with a secondary principalship, certainly the first in the district where I worked. How did this happen?

Being a principal was outstanding. We had, by far, the best secondary school in town. Most said it was our good clientele; some said it was because it was a new school. Still others offered other assessments. Of course, when someone else came along to be principal and things did not go as well, the clientele had changed, the school was not as new, and times were getting more difficult. There is no question that as a result of political advancement in society and our turning away from disciplinary concepts, it is indeed harder to work in the field of education today. It is my opinion, however, that things went so well during my time as principal because there were outstanding employees who worked together in a miraculous way. Kids did not want to disappoint us. Trust me, that is the truth. When they were sent to the office, most of the time they were apologetic. They were not apologetic because they thought they might get off. That would not happen and they knew it. They were sorry because they knew I would be disappointed, and I was. This began when I was an assistant principal and became even greater when I was principal. I mentioned earlier that it is also very unusual to become the principal where you have served as an assistant. If it is all marked up to coincidence, I have truly lived a life of coincidence. It would be interesting to have a statistician look at the many coincidences in my life and give an assessment of the probabilities. I believe it was all a miracle.

Three years after I became principal, a new superintendent was hired in the school district. He was in my school often. I was a nut about first impressions and keeping the school clean. It was my opinion that whoever walked in the door would judge us immediately by what they observed. We were friendly, organized, and attempted to be helpful to any visitor. Students were brainwashed to take pride in their school as well. For the most part, they were our best resource. We let students share in roles usually kept for adults in other schools. It is my opinion that we can live up to the expectations set for us if they are reasonable. Therefore, students had teacher duties in order to free teachers to do what they were hired to do. Students particularly liked to monitor hallways before school, and they performed wonderfully. It worked well for both students and teachers. Additionally, it allowed students to develop greater pride in their workplace, while at the same time to assist teachers and administrators. I must add that my secretary made me look good and kept us all on track. At any rate, for these many reasons, the new superintendent noticed our school and wanted me in central administration.

At the end of the first year under this superintendent, I was moved to the central administrative offices downtown. As detailed earlier, it was difficult in that I had my mother and her Alzheimer's to deal with. I still do not have an answer to sending my mother away, unless it simply points up my inability to handle the situation differently. I remain in prayer over this one.

The job, however, was another miracle of unusual proportion in my life. Here I was moving to the central office. There were so many others who had been in the district far longer than I. Why was I chosen? Additionally, my assignment was as director of fine arts. This entailed supervision of all band, choir, orchestra, art, and theatre arts programs. I had a degree major many years before in speech and drama, but *no* experience was attached. Where do you find credibility to work with some really outstanding professionals who can and do? Not only was life difficult at home with determining what I should do with mother, I had what seemed an insurmountable job ahead. The fine arts teachers in my school, although they were disappointed that I had to leave the position of principal, encouraged me in the new job. They were convinced that my leadership ability was more in need for the district fine arts programs than my do-ability. I tried to take their positive attitude and make it my own.

As school was nearing its start date, teachers were in staff-development sessions to prepare for the new school year. The time outlined for me to spend speaking with all fine arts personnel was one-half day. I prepared more for that four-hour speech than for any in my past experience.

The day arrived and I was in the appointed place for my encounter. As they came in, about sixty-five or seventy in my memory, it was obvious, particularly with the high school teachers, that it was a tell-me-why-you-are-our-boss time. Certainly, there was no verbal discourse on their part, but expressions and body language were far louder than any voice I had ever heard.

As the four-hour period of time moved forth, there were noticeable changes in my audience. By the end of the morning, only one person stood out as closed to the new direction. Fortunately, that was a person who became one of my greatest allies as time went by. It was amazing, however, how much these teachers gave to improve the fine arts programs. They were good teachers who needed leadership. I thank the Lord for their open minds. By the way, I thank God for this, another, miracle. As I look back at this time now, I realize it would have been impossible for the happenings to take place that did so. After a very short period of time, my credibility was on the rise.

Unfortunately, I thought, six months after being reassigned as director of fine arts, the superintendent moved me to an assistant superintendent position. I was to be supervisor for all principals. Principals had just begun to accept me in the fine arts position; now I was being moved into what was considered the most powerful position in the school district (other than superintendent). As it turned out, I supervised principals for almost ten years (including time with the superintendent who hired me and during my time as superintendent). After the first year or so, and particularly after my hitch in the personnel division, most principals respected my work. Many liked me and knew my entire life revolved around their work. A principal is, in my opinion, the most important person in a school district. It's a given that without a superintendent who guides the board and other central-office administrators to support and understand the principal position, a principal cannot be the best he can be. However, all things being equal, the principal molds the direction of a school. The greatest teacher in the world is not able to do his best without a district atmosphere and school environment conducive to learning.

Be all those things as they may, our school district soared for a time. It is my belief that principals were allowed to do a good job. For the most part, support was there for principals without which their jobs would have been even harder. It was an added time burden, but the principal had the last word in who was hired at his school. That practice was in place long before I became a teacher in the district. Every large school district of which I am aware, hires from the central office. Most school districts say they are saving their principals time. They are in actuality saving *themselves* time and effort rather than principals. It is my opinion that a campus is a family and the leader of that family is far better suited than the central office to know which teacher fits with others with whom they will work. The role of the central office should be to screen all applicants and send three or four of the best for the school to choose from. Principals or school committees can fine tune to hire the best choice for their needs.

It is my intent in this chapter to indicate where miracles occurred in my life. However, the temptation to "chase rabbits" relative to my past work takes over from time to time. It is probably obvious I have a passion for school leadership. It does fit together, however, in that my assignment to move into administration had to be a miracle. Who would have been assigned a job in an area like fine arts where they had no experience, let alone knowledge of music and art? At the end of six months, moving into an extremely powerful position in a city *very* insider motivated, was nothing short of a huge miracle. Additionally, I was a woman, and this was in the late 1980's where for the most part, women were not accepted in such powerful positions.

Nothing has been said about my drinking in this chapter; however, it is necessary to bring it up in the midst of all these exciting memories I've mentioned. While my work life became more and more hectic, my drinking became more difficult. It wasn't that I was drinking more; I was probably drinking less because there was just not enough time, but I was drinking every day, and I was drinking a lot. It was difficult to remember all that was on my plate at work every day. It was obvious to me I needed treatment, but where could I get treatment and not be found out? I prayed to the Lord over a rather long period of time. How long I do not remember, probably close to a year. I was at my wits end as to what I could do. One Saturday night in January, I spoke to the Lord and was ready to bite the bullet and go into treatment, whatever the personal cost. I had had a great deal to drink that day, no more than on some other occasions, but more than usual (around twenty drinks). After going to bed and sleeping only a short time, I awoke in a panic. My heart was racing, my chest felt like an elephant was sitting on it, and I was experiencing involuntary jerking in my extremities. It was one o'clock in the morning, and I did not know what to do. I asked God what in the world was going on. Should I wake up my roommate? Should I call a doctor? What should I do?

Each minute was an eternity. Thankfully, minutes turned into hours. By four o'clock that morning nothing had changed, and the Lord did not seem to be moving me toward doing anything. I decided I would wait until six or seven before I woke up my roommate to discuss what we might do. I was exhausted from all the shaking. I had ruled out a heart attack because nothing was intermittent. It was my fear that I had somehow become epileptic although that did not really fit either.

Just before six o'clock that morning, the shaking and rapid pulse stopped as quickly as it had begun. I fell asleep for almost two hours. When I awoke, I told my roommate about what happened in the night. Telling the story of what happened was just not the same as living it. The impact was not the same for others as it was for me.

As a result of all that happened on that cold January night, I was desperately afraid of alcohol. It was probably two or three weeks later that I realized it was all a miracle from God to stop my drinking. I heard stories that when people who consumed the quantity that I drank stopped drinking, they would go through a tough detoxification period. I experienced nothing.

Another miracle had come my way! It was nine years later before there was much desire for alcohol at all. On New Year's Eve before the year 2000, I experienced my first real desire for a drink. Today, I do desire a drink from time to time, and it takes willpower to say no. Additionally, I must also confess that there has been an occasion or two when my willpower has failed. The power alcohol has is a mystery to me. Getting high on Jesus is far more thrilling than any amount of alcohol can offer. Even so, the body is so weak! I will fight it on some level as long as I live.

Although alcohol played a devastating role for several years in my life, it is enough here to say that God took this person He loved and delivered her from its grip. I find it most amazing that the need was removed for the most part during the nine years after that fateful night. This was one event where I recognized the hand of God moving in my life. Had He not intervened when He did, I would have been unable to continue with my work. It appears it was not yet time for my work in education to end. At the time of this event, I had been at the central office three and a half years.

It was during the time that I wore so many hats that the Lord delivered me from alcohol. I presided over the divisions of administration, personnel, and assisted in developing the budget. When I look back now, I realize it was not possible to fulfill all the duties I had. It was true that I started my day at work around 6:30 in the morning and except for about an hour in the early evening to eat, I stayed at work until 10 or 10:30 each night. This was true day after day, week after week. It was wonderful!

Had I not been given strength and understanding of the jobs that needed to be done, it would have been impossible to take care of all that was on my plate. As I look back, it was not difficult at all. Certainly, it was work. It was long and tedious work, but I was in my element. I now believe there was a hand guiding me. For what purpose, I do not know. I may never know. I do believe it, however, with all my heart.

Without the varied experiences under the guidance of a most capable superintendent, I do not think the opportunity for my being superintendent would have arisen. As I write these words down, I know that if all of the timing had not been as it was, my life would have been far different. Again, I am amazed that this little kid who was shy, capable of less than admirable behavior, headed toward prison perhaps, and incapable of doing anything good was moved by the powerful hand of God in a direction only He understood. I sit here overwhelmed! The reader cannot grasp my awe.

Then there was retirement. Although I would not have chosen under earlier circumstances to retire when I did, I again believe it was the hand of God. I became frustrated with work, something unusual for me, and the state legislature changed the requirements for retiring, which allowed me full retirement if I chose. I had always said I would retire as soon as it was possible. Most people said it would be impossible for me to retire, that I was a workaholic and would be bored without my job. It was always my retort that I played as hard as I worked and would love to retire. My intent had always been to retire at age 57. Here I was 54 years old when the state rules changed. I pondered the situation.

There was a couple in our Sunday school class who introduced Anita and me to the book *Your Money or Your Life*. After reading the book, we decided we could manage our finances without working. Wow, this was good news, but I was not psychologically prepared. I had planned on three more years. What to do?

I offered prayer, prayer, and more prayer day after day. I was frustrated at work, but there were so many people I cared for. Also, there were the kids. How could the students get the best education possible without me watching over those who educated them? Each day I asked the Lord to make me rethink my decision, if I was making a mistake by retiring. Many times each day I would ask for it to be obvious if I should make the decision to stay. Day after day went by without my thinking that it was a mistake to leave, and although I was disappointed in one way, I was excited in another.

Without receiving information from the Lord to the contrary, I retired. It was indeed a new life. Wondering whether or not the decision had been the best one was not the least of my thoughts during the first year. The second year became easier as I let go of my previous work and the people I cared for there. As I reflected back, I realized the many joys I had experienced, and feelings of accomplishment and gratitude took over where only disappointments were felt during the first year.

My life as an educator had come to an end. I believe this was in accordance with God's perfect timing. There were four years between my retirement and the diagnosis of cancer. During those four years I had many opportunities that would not have come my way had I continued to work. Further, I would not have established a strong relationship with my church. Those sweet, sweet people have played a special part in this last year's journey. This past year in particular has been filled with permeating my mind with the Word, Christian television, prayer, and a wonderful life, far more fulfilling than any words can express. The greatest addiction one might have, in my opinion, is a continually growing desire for more of God.

Before I leave this chapter on miracles of God, I need to recount my move from the Baptist church. That move has played a significant part in my life since retirement. I believe different denominations are important. We need to study the Word and let the Lord speak to us concerning His will for our lives. I believe that He leads some of us in new directions at different times. Where He is in our lives, where we are in His will, and what that necessitates in needs, does not necessarily remain static throughout our life. Therefore, one denomination or another may be more fitting for us as individuals at a particular time in accordance with His leadership at that point in our lives. At one time (actually only a year ago if I am totally honest) I would not have accepted this thought at all. I believed the Baptist doctrine was the closest to correct and that was that! Everyone else missed the mark!

As stated before, I grew up a Baptist. I consider it a good thing that my family had been members of this denomination. It was good for me for many years, and I count it as positive that my upbringing was from a strict perspective. I was fifty years old before I veered from that doctrine in the church I attended, and although I have belonged to another denomination for the past several years, my basic beliefs continued in the Baptist stream of thought. I find it interesting that almost nine years ago I asked Anita about attending a particular Baptist church with me where I had been a member about fifteen years before. She agreed. Not giving much thought to the fact that in fifteen years many things change, we arrived at the church at 10:45 to attend what I believed would be a service beginning at 11:00. When we arrived, the parking lot was full, and there was no movement. I looked at the marquis and found that the service had begun at 10:30. Not wanting to arrive late, I suggested we attend another church and come to this one at another time.

Since it was agreeable with Anita to attend elsewhere, I quickly began to think of other churches in the neighborhood. It had been several years since I had lived in this town, and many things had changed. I suggested that another large church was located just down the freeway, but I was not sure of the denomination. She said she would attend any church other than a particular denomination she specified. I did not think it was the one she suggested as a no-no. We quickly drove down the freeway, and our timing was perfect. As we drove into the church parking lot, it was obvious that this was arrival time.

The sign signified that this was the First United Methodist Church. On arrival inside, we were greeted warmly by many, many people. We commented with one another that there was a "sweet, sweet, spirit in this place." It was obvious that this was a wonderful, spirit-filled church. Actually, I had never been in a fellowship where I experienced this special feeling, except while attending some crusades when the altar call was given and thousands of people moved forward. Here, we were simply sitting, waiting for the service to begin.

It was only a short time before the service began. Quickly, we realized this was a charismatic fellowship. Neither one of us had experienced this before. It was not like the usual charismatic churches where they were speaking in tongues and other more indicative behavior of what some may identify with the charismatic movement. From time to time someone would lift his hands in praise, but that was all, other than a great deal of clapping. It would not have been comfortable for me to raise my arms, but observing others was not uncomfortable at all. In fact, I loved the fellowship, the music, and the spirit that I could not put my finger on. It was unlike any feeling I had previously experienced in church. The music made me feel transported to a heavenly choir. Anita experienced the same things. We continued to attend this church until four years ago when we retired and moved to a small town.

One of the most difficult things about retirement was leaving this church. It was not in the same city where I worked, but it was close enough to drive there on Sundays. When we retired, we moved too far away to continue attending there on a regular basis. It had become apparent to us both, however, that we no longer were of the Baptist persuasion, although basic beliefs remained. I think Anita had realized this many years before while married to a Baptist minister where she was a vital participant in his work. It is understandably expected for a spouse to remain in the same denomination.

Retired, we resumed our search for the right church. Although I thought myself no longer aligned with as much Baptist theology as I previously believed, I did not know what exact beliefs I thought should change. We knew we wanted to be in a fellowship where there was borderline charismatic behavior and less dogmatic theology. We visited church after church of every denomination except one and did not find a church that either of us was moved to join. This continued week after week without success. We continued to pray about it and spoke with one of the ministers in the Methodist church where we had attended. We continued to drive well over an hour each way from time to time just to be fed. There was a huge hole in our lives. Where were we to worship? The answer just did not come. The minister with whom we spoke encouraged us to attend even the really charismatic denominations and see if the Lord led us there. He did not.

We had just about given up. There was a Methodist church on the downtown square of the town where we had moved, and we decided to join there. It did not meet the criteria we thought we were looking for, but we needed to get on with our Christian work. The people were nice, and we did not have a better solution than to join there. In fact, one Sunday morning we decided to make the move. However, on that particular morning, the minister announced that he was being transferred. His transfer was not a problem, but his attitude was unusual. We could not put our finger on the problem, but we decided to wait.

That afternoon while reading the newspaper, I noticed a picture of a lady who was identified as the music director of First Christian Church (Disciples of Christ) in the town. She was a well-known manager of the historic opera house and an extremely talented musician. We were both intrigued that she was leading music in a local church. It happened to be a church we had not visited. It was a small church in a location we had somehow missed.

On the following Sunday we attended the church. It was a small fellowship of around two hundred and fifty. The music was very good and the minister had something to say. We went back for several weeks and found the members to be friendly and encouraging. It was a more formal service than we were accustomed to. We met with the pastor to discuss joining. He was most receptive, and we joined on the following Sunday. We began singing in the choir and became very involved in every area of the church.

All this discussion about the churches has been to point out what I believe to be another miracle. I believe the Lord intended for us to visit the First United Methodist Church the day we intended to visit the Baptist church but had gone at the wrong time. That fellowship took me to a new level of group worship I had never experienced before. It led to a deeper relationship with the Lord than I had previously experienced. It is impossible to put on paper all I know has been a result of this experience. This past year would have been far different without that occurrence.

It is just as miraculous that one Sunday afternoon while looking through the newspaper a picture was seen and a church visited that would have otherwise been overlooked. That church is our current church home. It is the church that saw me through my cancer diagnosis and resulting concerns. It is the church that just happened to have a previous long-time chaplain from a large cancer center in the United States as the interim minister at the exact time I needed him. I find it interesting, as well, that the interim minister was replaced by another interim minister after a short period of time because of his health problems. He was there just long enough to minister to me in a desperate time of need.

Without experiencing this changing of churches, my life would have taken a different turn. My beliefs (which I will detail in the next chapter) have dramatically changed. My earlier beliefs were right for me then. My current beliefs are right for me now. Without these changes, this book would not be written. Without these changes I do not believe the Lord would have set me apart to do this work.

BURDENED TO WRITE

Just before my six-month appointment with the surgeon after the tumor was removed, I experienced a tinge of anxiety, although for the most part I believed a healing had taken place. By all accounts I should have been feeling quite sick. Most information on the Internet provided a dismal prognosis because after this cancer had been touched, it spread quite rapidly. It appeared to me that all of the professionals I had seen since the cancer diagnosis were expecting bad news as well.

During the six months I waited to find out, I had experienced a relationship with God unparalleled in my life. The "lightning experience and angel encounter" in my teenage years had been miniscule compared with the plethora of experiences over this time. It seemed the Lord was always there when I needed Him. Whether He spoke through what we would call coincidental occurrences, the Word, other people, nature, or His Spirit, it seemed there was constant communication.

One such experience occurred three days following surgery, when I was in bed recuperating and before realization that the tumor was malignant. It was 8:25 P.M. on the Friday evening prior to

Labor Day. I noticed my aging dog walking in an extremely wobbly manner toward his doggie door. When he got to the door, he fell, got up, fell again, got up and stood there unsteadily. I called to Anita to come see what was wrong. By the time she got to the room, he had made it outside. She went out and said he looked like he was having a stroke. This was my baby! I was ill; how could God let him be having problems now! It was Labor Day weekend, and his vet was the owner of the clinic. What would the chances be that he was the one on call? Probably slim to none!

I called the answering service for the clinic and asked who was on call. Unbelievably, it was my vet. I asked her to please have the doctor call me soon. At 8:30 P.M. the doctor called back. It had been five minutes since it all began. The vet was at a party but asked how long it would take to get the dog to his office. Anita said she could be there in about ten minutes. He said it would take him about the same. Anita picked up the dog (about 55 pounds) and got him into the car. Anita with Towser, and the vet all arrived at the office at 8:40 P.M. Anita called me at 8:50 P.M. and said Towser was not responding to I.V. Valium, which indicated he had a brain lesion. The vet gave a grim prognosis. He was too old for surgery, but I was having a hard time letting him go. I said it was necessary to put him to sleep. At 9:00 P.M. Anita called and said it was done.

Wow! My baby was gone! How was I going to handle it? Additionally, I had been told not to cry because of all the packing in my sinuses and nasal area. There was lots of packing. The tumor had been vascular, my nose had been broken, and my head felt like a large beach ball. The swelling was quite noticeable as well. Why now, God? Why now?

Four days after having put Towser to sleep, I began hemorrhaging and was admitted into the hospital for several days. The hospital was in a city too far away for Anita to leave me to go back to Towser, had he been living. Towser had separation anxiety and would have become quite ill with me away, and I would have been beside myself with worry as well. Our vet had been on duty the Friday evening of Towser's need, Labor Day weekend. Towser was in his state of anxiety only thirty-five minutes. It was probably also good that I was not with him when he died. God gave me His answer. It had been a miracle. His timing is always *perfect*!

His timing was also perfect when it came to deciding about cancer treatment two or three weeks after the Towser incident. It was obvious that He was telling me not to have treatment. As I look back on it now, it seems unreal! How often do we seek counsel from physicians about a diagnosis of cancer after surgery, then deny treatment? That is unheard of! I cannot imagine it as I sit here typing. Usually when a health concern comes up, I ask the physician or seek counsel from Anita (a retired health-care professional) concerning what I should do. This time, I asked the Lord, and He gave me a most unusual answer—unusual as far as my previous history would have dictated.

After the decision was made not to have treatment, I was very comfortable with that decision. I look back now, and it all seems like a dream. That was only a year ago. Oh so many things have taken place during this year! In mid-October of last year, about a year ago today, I was requesting God to speak to me, to say something more as I opened my Bible. I was doing fine with my decision not to have treatment. I was healing from my surgery and was feeling quite well. I felt close to the Lord but felt at loose ends. He was gracious to me as always, and as I opened my Bible (anywhere it fell was the deal) to Romans 8 and my eyes fell on verse 11. Whatever the translation I use at the time is the one accepted. On this occasion I was using the New International Version (NIV). I take literal meanings of text whether or not the meaning in context is different. In the case of this verse, in context it means that our bodies will have life renewed after death. However, the literal interpretation of this verse in the NIV without context in verse 11b says "he who raised Christ from the dead will also *give life to your mortal bodies* through his Spirit, who lives in you." Life to my "mortal body." Could this mean I was going to live awhile? I wondered. Some may say this is stretching it since a literal meaning is used rather than in context. They may be correct, but God and I have done it this way for a long time.

At any rate, it was six or seven weeks post-surgery, and this said to me that God was not through with me yet! Although my anxiety level heightened to a degree just before the surgeon performed an endoscopy approximately four months later, I held this verse tightly against my heart until the day of proof.

Another Scripture I looked back to for comfort came about six months before surgery when I had asked God to speak with me in the same manner (open the Bible, give me a Scripture). At that time, I was having a difficult time with my life in general. My mother having had Alzheimer's provided a fifty-percent chance for my ending up with the same disease. Not long after her death many years before, I had pondered on the possibilities of my having that dreaded disease in future years. I imagined I was experiencing memory loss, too (the ravings of an alcoholic). That had been about thirteen years before this current plea for a message. Not all of that thirteen years had been spent worrying about contracting Alzheimer's, but it was always in the back of my mind, I suppose. Last spring a year ago, Anita was involved in her family's decision to place her dad in a nursing home as a result of his dementia. Her mother had valiantly taken care of him as long as she could, but her health began to fail as a result of losing sleep caring for him. Anita, having the expertise with health care and nursing home facilities, took the lead in securing a suitable place for her dad. It brought back memories for me, and as a result, I was at loose ends. For reasons I'll not explain, my fear of Alzheimer's became unbearable. Of course, as is usual for me, I did not tell anyone. Pressures built up and life at home became difficult as well.

It was in this desperation that I appealed to the Lord. It was certainly unknown to me at that time, that six months in the future I would have a malignant tumor removed. Having a malignant tumor removed put a whole new light on Alzheimer's disease. How quickly our perspectives change! Be all that as it may, I had asked the Lord for a message that day six months prior to my illness, and the Williams New Testament Translation opened to Philippians 4. My eyes fell on some very familiar Scripture in verses 4–7 printed below.

> By the help of the Lord always keep up the glad spirit; Yes, I will repeat it, keep up the glad spirit. Let your for-bearing spirit be known to everybody. The Lord is near. Stop being worried about anything, but always, in prayer and entreaty, and with thanksgiving, keep on making your wants known to God. Then through your union with Christ Jesus, the peace of God, that surpasses all human thought, will keep guard over your hearts and thoughts.

In the middle of the following October, after fleecing for the Scripture (two months after surgery when I again asked the Lord to speak with me), while reading the passage in Romans, I remembered this message from Philippians. I once more looked at these verses with greater intensity. They had been most comforting the spring prior, and now they provided new meaning. Whether or not looking at them again was a fair part of my fleecing, I do not know. I just know I thought of them as I looked at Romans. It seemed to me the Lord could be telling me through both passages that He was not finished with me yet. At this point I was feeling great peace. I did not necessarily think I would be physically healed, but I believed I was healed in some context. Whether the Lord was physically healing me, going to rapture me (the Lord is near in Philippians 4:5b), or He was going to take me home, I did not know. Whatever happened, I was experiencing God's peace. If He chose to take me home, I wanted to be the best witness who had ever lived yet who was soon to die.

Later in October, I did something that was a real stretch for me. Although I had branched out in my theology and even embraced mild charismatic services while earlier attending the Methodist church, I decided to attend a crusade led by one who some think a quack. Although I did not think his salvation was fraudulent, I did not know how much theatrical involvement there was in his crusades.

In the early 1990's, while browsing in a bookstore for something to read, I came across a book by an author I had never heard of. His name was Benny Hinn, and the book was *Good Morning Holy Spirit*. It looked like an interesting book, and I bought it. Having never heard of this author, I had no preconceived opinion of its worth. The Lord used the book to speak with me in a mighty way. Over the last ten years I read the book several times to energize myself in the spirit from time to time.

So, after having developed my own opinion that he was a spirit-filled Christian who God used in my life, I was open to test my opinion beyond the book. This Benny Hinn guy was conducting a crusade in Shreveport, Louisiana, and Anita and I decided to go. My body was feeling well for the most part although all the swelling resulting from my nose having been broken (I had had a deviated septum) was not completely gone. We made reservations at a hotel (it was difficult to get a hotel: most were taken by others coming to the crusade) and began our journey. I found it interesting that it was hard to find a room just because some preacher was coming into town, but that was what they said.

What a shock! We stood in line for hours before time for the service in order to get a seat! It was a good thing we decided to find out where the center was where he would preach in several hours and saw that the line had already begun. Otherwise, we would have arrived much later and not gotten a seat, after driving five or six hours from home to get to this crusade. We quickly went back to our room, changed clothes, and returned. About three hours later, the service was to begin.

We went inside the coliseum that seated about 15,000 people and it was almost full, three hours early! What in the world! We found a place to sit next to a nice looking thirty-something year old African-American gentleman who was affable. We soon struck up a conversation with him. He was a Pentecostal minister whose wife was singing in the crusade choir. This gentleman had practiced with the choir the previous evening but felt the Lord had told him to sit with the masses when he arrived that day. Further, he said the Lord had told him to sit in the seat where he was. In the faiths I have been a party to in my life, we didn't talk about the Lord in this way. We might think from time to time that the Lord has led us in a particular direction, but to say "God said to me" was not part of my understanding. I accepted what he said as well as I could and continued on with the conversation.

As time went by and the service began, the atmosphere was charged with excitement. The music was as beautiful as I had ever heard, and there was not one seat empty in the coliseum! Fifteen thousand people were singing and praising the Lord. Although I did not participate with the hands in the air behavior, I knew the Lord was there. What a spirit-filled group of people this was! There were many outside who could not be accommodated. I had to admit it was heartwarming to see so many people on fire for God.

Partway into the service, the gentleman beside me asked if he could pray for me. I had told him that a cancerous tumor had been removed less than two months prior. It was a beautiful prayer that lasted for what seemed to be a long time. My body did not experience anything different, but tears streamed down my face to the point of embarrassment. Tears began to flow down his face as well, as we stood arm in arm while he prayed.

What an experience! The crusade continued for three services in a two-day period. Each service lasted three or four hours. My life was transformed. On the last evening of the crusade, the audience was asked to "image" the Lord. I thought of a waterfall and brook where I saw Jesus, hugged Him and began to feel a warmth throughout my chest. What that signified, I do not know, but I felt it had some kind of significance. I have, or had, two leaky valves in my heart. I have wondered if they, too, are healed. I do not know, but I am sure the Lord intended for me to attend those services. As a side note, I've tried to e-mail the gentleman sitting beside me but have never received an answer. Was he really at the crusade? Maybe I've read too many angel books!

Thanksgiving and Christmas (2001) came and went. Time continued to pass, moving toward the six-month visit with the surgeon for an endoscopy in February. On the night preceding my visit with the doctor, I had a dream. Seldom do I remember dreams, but I heard someone speak on Christian television some time before who said you could do many things to try to remember your dreams. I made some attempts with little success. However, on this occasion, I remembered my dream. In fact, on several occasions last March and April, I remembered my dreams. I find it interesting because for the past six months since that time I have not remembered any dreams.

On the night before my visit, I had a dream that I was set apart. In the dream there was a really bright sun. Also, I thought I had some awake visions during the dream of three huge bomb blasts in the distance. I used my Bible concordance to look up every *set apart* I could find, then I looked up *bright sun*, and then *three huge mounds of fire and smoke*. I found that every time I could find *set apart* it referred to belonging to God. In Malachi and Isaiah, I found that a bright sun signified love and Jesus. In Joel, I found that fire and smoke were signs of God's presence. I then interpreted it to mean that God had set me apart for something through the love of

Jesus with the presence of God in three (Father, Son and Holy Spirit).

When I went to the appointment with the surgeon after having the dream, although I must admit there was some wonder whether or not he would find new tumor growth, I was armed and ready. What a wonderful dream I had, what a wonderful Lord!

As detailed in the first chapter, when I saw the physician and he performed the endoscopy, there was a really long pause before he told me it was clean as a whistle. He said a bit later in the visit, "It will be interesting if nothing else shows up and I wanted to take your body apart." Only, right this minute as I type these words I notice he said "apart." I wonder if this has anything to do with the *set apart*? It's something new to think about. Wow!

In addition to this visit with the surgeon, as earlier discussed, I went to my ophthalmologist the following day, and she informed me that my right optic nerve was "pink, pulsating and very healthy looking." It was at this point that I really began to believe the Lord was choosing to heal me physically.

The other five dreams from last spring (2002) came over a short period of time. The night of April 6, I had a dream and awoke feeling frantic because I couldn't remember anything. I felt I was supposed to remember something. I asked the Lord for help, and the words, "You were looking for a place to stay" came to my mind. I did not, nor do I know what they mean, but I was no longer panicked when the words came to me. On the night of April 7, I had a dream that "God leads His dear children along," words to a great old song which are self-explanatory. And, on April 9, I dreamed something about three o'clock. I do not know whether it was in the morning or evening, but I thought about *timing*. About 3:00 P.M. Jesus said "Why have You forsaken me; it is finished; and unto You I commit my spirit." I wonder what this meant. Perhaps I am placing too much emphasis on dreams, but I have come to believe that God indeed speaks to us in more ways than I had earlier thought. I don't want to miss a word!

Next to the last dream from that group came on April 15. My memory was only for words. They were, "When the nails are out, hammer them back in." Only in Colossians did I find anything that might be important. Colossians 2:14 in the Williams New Testament states ". . . canceled the note that stood against us, with its requirements, and has put it out of our way by nailing it to the cross." What a deal! And last, on April 28 during a nap, I dreamed about rowing a lifeboat. I have been told that any time you dream about a mode of transportation, you are dreaming about a life-change. Oh, what a life change I have experienced over this past year! In the following chapter, I will try to put on paper some of the theological changes I have made over this past year.

Somewhere about the time I was experiencing these dreams, I kept feeling that I was truly healed of cancer and that I was to do something as a result. What? What in the world could I do? I had told my Sunday school class about all that had transpired. They were given a blow-by-blow description of every comment made and every feeling felt. What else could I do? They responded favorably, and I knew it was being discussed by many throughout the church, but I continued to feel there was something else.

Then in July of 2002, only a few months after all the dreams, someone was speaking with me about a Scripture. My memory is that it had something to do with prophesy. I am not sure, but I thought it was. I "accidentally" turned to Psalm 118:17. It says, "I will not die, but I will live to tell what the Lord has done." I was stunned! I read it over and over. Then, I realized I had looked up the wrong Scripture. However, when I looked at Psalm 108:17, there was not a seventeenth verse. Not remembering who had mentioned the Scripture, I have been unable to find out what I was told to look up. I only saw what I believe the Lord had me look up. I know it seems unbelievable that I looked up this Scripture by mistake, but it is the truth! How often do things arise that we just can't believe because everything must fit into coincidence? Far too much in the life of this fifty-eight-year-old sinner of sinners has happened that cannot be explained other than by miracles which were individually put off as coincidences as they happened. It took a lethal form of cancer and intervention by the living God to show how He sets us apart by His grace! I believe we each have a mission from God, just waiting for our recognition. We have all experienced miracles in our lives and called them coincidences. What grief, what grief we give our Lord!

My life is the last life that God should cleanse, but He told us that, "His ways are not our ways." It was hard for me to accept that the almighty God was wanting something from *me*, but I continued to feel a need to do something. When I read Psalm 118:17 at one point and asked the Lord who or what I could do to tell, I realized that a book about my life might be what was necessary. Telling about this last year would be wonderful, other than the fact that I am an old science teacher who, except for working on college papers, a thesis, and a dissertation, always ran the other way from writing. Also, there were too many really ugly things in my life that I did not want to remember, even for myself, much less put them out there for anyone to see. How would my family feel? What would friends think? It is really scary to put your life down on paper. True, you have many memories that come to mind that you leave out. You remember them just the same.

Burdened to tell. Those are the words that kept coming to my mind. I told the Lord I would make an attempt to write a book after the check-up at the end of a year, after proof was there from an MRI. It was only a month away.

Tests were back, no sign of cancer. I was burdened to write. Does that mean I will live a long time? I do not know what it means except I believe I will live long enough to write this book. What He has for me after that only He knows. I do know this past year would have turned out differently if treatment had been a choice. It was not. Praise God! There are so very many things that have taken place (coincidences?) this past year that have been incredible, and taken together, have made God's mission for me undeniable.

This past year has been the most wonderful of my life. It has been filled with miracle upon miracle and an unparalleled closeness with the Lord. It was not the only time I experienced miracles or a closer walk; however, it was simply the most spectacular. I am convinced God leads His dear children along sometimes when they do not even know it. It has certainly been true for me.

Chapter 16

A CHANGE IN THEOLOGY

Over the past eight or nine years, my theological belief structure has moved in a different direction. The law-oriented upbringing and continuation until after my fiftieth birthday made my movement toward center unusual perhaps. It is my opinion that the refinement in my beliefs has been through guidance from God.

For the past thirty years, I have been a student of Bible prophesy. It is my opinion that anyone who truly takes the time to study prophesy with an open mind develops a foundation for belief in the Bible itself. Reading commentaries on prophetic Scripture, written by individuals God appears to have chosen for unfolding the mysteries, was a beginning for me. Listening to the Holy Spirit within us as we read the prophetic literature, both in the Bible and as discerned by others, as well as digging through the book of Revelation goes hand in hand as well. Nothing has changed the beliefs that developed during my thirty-year study. There have only been refinements over these last eight or nine years. In fact, I believe the Lord has revealed even more to me about prophesy during this time. His Word says we are not to be afraid because He is coming soon. Soon to us? I do not know. It certainly was not soon on our timetable considering the date He provided the information. What I do know is that His timing is always perfect. It appears to be so in Scripture, and as I review my life, it appears the same. Whenever it is, I say, "Come!" We may not know the day or the hour, but He tells us to know the signs of the time.

Some may discount the book of Revelation, but if we believe Isaiah, Ezekiel, Daniel, and many of the other prophetic books, as well as information Jesus gave in the gospels, we believe He is coming back. Most Christians say they believe it. If they really believe it, they are looking up. It concerns me that we often make people fear those things that surround an end. An end simply marks a new beginning. What a gift!

Although my belief about a catching away, a tribulation, and a thousand-year reign of Christ on the earth have remained intact, many ideas unrelated to prophesy have changed. I think my beliefs are a result of hours of prayer, Bible study, and what I believe is enlightenment from God over this past year. Most changes have occurred over the past six months. When your beliefs change as much as mine have in such a short time, it creates great excitement, while at the same time promoting great introspection. One day in prayer I was "given" the statement, "I can believe only as much as my ignorance will allow." Wow, that was profound! I could not have thought of that. Where did it come from? I spoke earlier about people in some faiths saying, "God said this to me and God said that to me." My frame of reference only had God speaking to me when I fleeced Him. I also picked up somewhere that you shouldn't fleece. Oh my, I was bad again! I am sorry, but I just had to know.

Here I was, thinking I understood what was meant by "God said this to me!" I admit, I have no other explanation. I also have to admit that I am hardheaded enough that I do not think I could be believing this unless it happened to me personally. Further, were I reading this about someone else, I would probably think the cancer had invaded the brain for sure! I cannot possibly let the reader understand how foreign many of the things I am saying, or going to say, would have been to me over my adult life, even one year ago. It more than frightens me to put it into print. I do not want to. Please God, don't make me tell!

Although much of the meanness of my early years did not make it into print, just about everything I *have* been burdened to tell has been hard to write. Recounting the miracles in my life was wonderful. In fact, realizing the thread of the miraculous that has woven through my life is something for which I thank God. He has been with me through it all. He was there with every wart I experienced. He has removed them all! I give praise! My outside is as rotten as ever, but my inside is white as snow.

One of the things I have realized is how much fear I have lived with in my life. I always passed it off by saying that I came from a family of worriers. My parents were worriers before me, and I simply was carrying on the tradition. We know at a head level, how fear is simply a lack of faith. I knew that but had not internalized it. My fears of fear and anxiety have been with me since I was a small child. My fear for my mother dying began when I was six years old. That is the earliest fear I remember. It was a fear that carried an underlying feeling that came out in full force when my grandfather (her dad) died. I was twenty-one years old at the time. Then, I became paralyzed with fear for my mother's death. I do not remember what I thought my fear might be about; I only know I became suicidal. That was the beginning of my pill path that lasted about fifteen years. I have experienced fear whether it was realistic or not. Fearing for my mother's death from the time I was six years old until she had a heart attack during my thirty-eighth year equates to a long thirty-two years of wasted worry time! The Lord did something for me when she had the heart attack that released the great fear I had for her death. After the heart attack, I told my mother I loved her for the very first time. That probably seems impossible to the reader; it seems impossible to me. It has been easier for me to tell those with whom I am comfortable that I love them and give hugs since that occurred back in the early 1980's, but before that time, I ran from any demonstration of love. If I didn't demonstrate love, maybe I would not be hurt when it died!

The fear of death I had for those I loved died with mother's heart attack. It was certainly not the end of my worry nature: it simply began a new chapter with a different twist. Most of my fears became phobias that I was able to keep others from knowing about. Fear for fear and anxiety are all encompassing and are perhaps worst of all. In our humanity we all have our fears, but they indeed result from lack of faith. It has only been in this past year that I have recognized and faced my deepest fears. My deepened relationship with God over this past year has pointed out many of my shortcomings and given me hope for their demise. He is the answer! It takes continued growth in Him and trust for His guidance.

Why is it so hard to believe that God speaks to us? If we believe the Bible, we believe God spoke to people for thousands of years in both Old and New Testament times. We believe He performed miracles, too. But for some reason, He stopped talking and He stopped performing miracles. He even *appeared* to some many years ago. Our belief is so small; He certainly would not appear to us! Actually, as I look at it now, it would not make sense for Him to communicate and heal for five or so thousand years and then stop! If that is so, He probably never did any of those things at all. If that is so, the Bible is a lie. If that is so, we need to give it up! We might as well: we don't even believe in angels. I had an angel story for forty years that I slapped God in the face with, as I would not even think about it!

There is no question today that I would stake my life on the fact of God's reality. We have *so* many doubts. Even the best of Christians have doubts, in one way or another. It is part of living in this world. The Bible says the world was given to Satan for a time. This is just a part of it. If we did not have doubts, we would *not* live the lives we live. We would be feeding the poor, serving our neighbors, and going door to door with the good news that Christ died for us. Think about it—it's true! Every church would have lots of money and never beg for workers. As I look at it, I do not think we really believe. We give lip service just in case. We do those things we think might be enough, just in case it is not all a fabrication of some deranged minds long ago! No, maybe we want to hang on to it so we can prove to ourselves that we are just a little better than someone else. Sure, we're really all right, deep down. If it is true, a loving God will certainly take *us*. We do not do those really bad things. Surely it will all come out all right.

Chapter 17

LAW OR LOVE

Where does greatest truth lie, in law or in love? My earlier beliefs centered on law. I was more interested in all the things that were thou shalt not! Where the Bible says that Jesus fulfilled the law, I wanted to pass right over it. The Bible also tells us not to remove one thing written. I believe the Bible tells me I have spent far too much time looking at the Old Testament law, with far too little time in the New Testament grace. The Old Testament is filled with grace, but I (and others), often see too much law rather than grace there as well. That was the same problem with the Pharisees. Remember, also, they had Jesus crucified! We follow in the same path as they! Will Jesus see many of us any differently from the way He saw them? It may be something to think about.

Without God's grace, there is no hope. That is truth, but that is not the problem. I see the problem as each of us wanting to play God. We say that is not so; however, listen to many often well-meaning Christians as they judge. They may predicate what they say with, "Now I don't want to judge, but . . ." Don't want to judge! We think if we say these magic words that our inappropriate behavior (sin?) will be overlooked! We have made up our own rules about sin. We have developed our own hierarchy of sin. We want to be told, and tell others, just how desperately bad *they* are! Is that in keeping with the way Jesus taught?

Jesus gave us two laws. First, He said we were to love God completely; secondly, we were to love our neighbor as ourselves. My thoughts are that we do not love God as we should. We place just about everything before God. If all else rests on this first requirement, I wonder how many of us are in real trouble to start with?

Recently, I spent a great deal of time thinking about the second command. I thought about my neighbors and how I felt about them. It seemed to me that I loved my household, my relatives, and my close friends more than the rest of society. How could I love my neighbor as myself? There are some people I would die for instead of trying to save myself first, but that would not be everyone. It may be a "no brainer" for my reader, but it appeared to me in prayer one day that to love my neighbor was simply a command to do unto my neighbor what I would choose for him to do for me. That's right, to invoke the Golden Rule (Luke 7:31) with my neighbor. As simple as this is, it took some thinking on my part to believe I understood the second command. It is true, however, when we invoke the Golden Rule with our fellow man, we will not take their husband, wife, or property, or do anything that would be of harm to them. Additionally, if we love our neighbor as ourselves, we will feed the hungry, care for the needy, and tell others about Jesus' desire that "none should perish." The remainder of the Ten Commandments rest on the first two. Jesus gave Christians the two commandments to live by, whereas the Jews were given the original ten through Moses. Some may say the difference is small; I think it quite significant.

It appears to me that when we get too caught up in law, we cannot properly fulfill what is required by love. We are to love. Jesus did. He set the example for us—at least He tried to. I spent much of my life wanting to use law and love where each was of greatest benefit to what I wanted to be right. It at least appears that is true. Those sins I was not involved deeply with I chose to be the bad ones, while those I lived in were not nearly as bad as the other sins. In fact, I knew I must be closer to God than those who did those other awful things! We pick and choose what we want to judge, based on our own shortcomings!

Were we to look through the Bible as a total entity, we would find that a hierarchy of sin would place idol worship on top, with all others distantly behind and equal. In today's society, we usually place murder highest in our hierarchy and probably homosexuality somewhere near number two. In the Bible hierarchy, idol worship (which basically reveals our lack of God) is our worst sin. In John 16:9 Jesus says, "The world's sin is unbelief in me." That makes sense since Jesus said the greatest commandment was to love the Lord our God with all our heart, mind, and strength first. However, in our world we worship what money can buy far more than we worship God. Anyone who thinks differently needs only to look at his checkbook and see where the money goes. Does it go for things we want (after necessities), or does it go to the church, to feed the poor, and to evangelize the world? Most of us spend far more on our loved ones or ourselves than in those areas that Jesus might choose. He said that when we give to someone in need, we are giving to Him. That is what He said! How much do we do that? There is proof enough right here that most of us have a serious problem we give *little or no* thought to. Additionally, what about our spare time? Do we read the Bible, or do we pursue other interests? If we were on fire for God, we would be seen reading our Bibles in every spare moment. We would be driven to study His Word!

Much is mentioned in the Bible about lying, as well. We glaze over that, too. In our daily lives, we lie unless we are locked up in a closet somewhere. The way we listen when someone else speaks, the way we sometimes shake our heads in agreement when really we disagree is a lie. We want acceptance in this world so much we try not to make waves. We pass it off, saying there is no reason to hurt someone unnecessarily. There is no reason to cause a disagreement when unnecessary. These may not be of any consequence we say, but they are still lies. Let's face it: we are liars! We say it was just "a little white lie" and give it no more thought. This may or may not be earth-shaking news, but it came to me in prayer and seemed to be His answer to some of my questioning about judging. We are all guilty. Why do we not just accept each other as we are and show love.

How many times have we seen someone profess faith in Christ and expect that person to make specific changes in his life immediately? The expectations we should have are that they show love for God and for others. Instead, I have seen those who condemn their spiked hairdos, the rings in their nose, the wrong kinds of clothes, etc. We place judgment on what they will outwardly do or not do, rather than what takes place inwardly. We just cannot seem to let them grow in the Lord. Why not encourage them to read Scripture, to pray, and provide them with *loving* guidance, rather than try to clean them up on the outside? We mix up religion with Christianity and therefore turn away the unsaved and newly saved.

Kids, in particular, may need time to be moved to change outward behavior. They have friends to consider. We often disregard things that are unimportant to us or things we do not understand. It takes *time* to grow in Christ. What about us? It appears we who want to impose our own demands need as much growth as the new Christian! We remain babes for a long time unless we let the Spirit lead us through study and prayer. When left alone, some kids make changes in due time. Sometimes, granted, changes are not made, but that should be left alone, too. We often wonder why kids do not listen to adults. Often, we as adults preach the inward while judging the outward. Kids notice! We tell them to come as you are, but the minute they come, we tell them, "These are the changes you must make." Why can we not leave it with God? I think it is because we want to be the judge. You know, this makes me wonder if many of us simply give lip service to God. Why do we need Him? With Christians appearing to be negative and judgmental, why would *anyone* want to be one?

For many, as mentioned earlier, second on the hierarchy of bad is homosexuality. It is second only to murder. You say, "Look in the Bible. Look in the Bible." I have looked in the Bible. I see a lot of other things mentioned as well—things like lying, for instance, which is mentioned far more and I see us all as liars. We blame homosexuality for everything because homosexuals are an easy target. We do not care how many homosexuals hate us, so we go after them. AIDS is always mentioned in connection with homosexuality. Drug abusers and heterosexual promiscuity are guilty for the AIDS epidemic as well, but we only want to talk about the homosexual, saying it is the most prevalent cause. Why do we not talk about homosexual promiscuity? Because most of us think all homosexuals are promiscuous anyway. We place God's fervent wrath on something *we* want to blast, while knowing or caring very little about these aberrations of humanity.

Having people think my lifestyle to mean that I had sex with girls, I came to recognize more about "gayness" than I really care to know. Contrary to what many may believe, there are gay people who love God. Many gays live in the closet or are married to survive. When they also live a gay lifestyle on the side, pain is spread in many, many directions. Also, those people who are just not the marrying kind, who seek a companion because they do not want to live alone, also experience discrimination whether gay or not.

We think pedophilia and homosexuality are synonymous terms. They are not. Most homosexuals are only interested in adult partners. Some perhaps become involved in errant behavior with children, but most sexual-abuse cases in children are a result of heterosexual people, not homosexual. It is possible for those of any persuasion to become criminally involved with children, but to think it more often homosexual than heterosexual is incorrect. Often, homosexual men are extremely compassionate and gentle with children. Pedophiles are a different matter. They prey on children and exhibit criminal behavior. Unfortunately, we treat them all the same.

To lump all groups into one is just about as judgmental and incorrect as is possible. When criminal behavior is the problem, prosecute. Otherwise, it belongs to God just like anything else we consider wrong observed in others. We use the slogan "What Would Jesus Do?" and were we to review His behavior and teaching, I think we would see that He would handle this topic far differently from the way we do. It might be that someone without sin should "cast the first stone." What is sin for one, may or may not be sin for another; *we* want to decide. Why can't we let Him?

Whatever the infraction, we want to pick and choose those things we want to say are really bad sins. The Pharisees did the same when they complained bitterly with Jesus that His disciples "eat and drink with such scum" (Luke 5:30b). Jesus said in Luke 5:32, "I have come to call sinners to turn from their sins, not to spend my time with those who think they are already good enough." Is it not wonderful, He stated "who think they are already good enough?" My concern is that we are sometimes those who think we are too good to reach out to everyone, regardless of who they are or what they have done. Our behavior would say so. This passage on the Pharisees sounds like us, as it is we who want to tell others what is good and bad. What happens when we invite people to church with us who good folks do not want to be a part of their fellowship because of the way they dress? Oh, how we judge to make ourselves look just.

Again in Luke 6:2b, the Pharisees point out that grain is not to be harvested on the Sabbath; therefore, Jesus' disciples had broken the law. Jesus disagreed. He was accused many times of not obeying the law. Oh, I think there must be a lesson here! In each instance, it appears Jesus was showing us picture after picture of ourselves, but He has not gotten a response from this generation just as He did not then. No, no, I am wrong. He got a response; they crucified Him! We haven't changed; we crucify Him every day. The Pharisees looked for things Jesus did against the law. Do we do the same to others? Is it because we want to think ourselves better than they, because we want to play or be God, or is it that we are truly evil? To whom do we *really* belong? Each of us who professes to be a Christian needs to take a long, hard look! Do we really believe the truth? It does not appear that we *really* do. In Luke 11:35, Jesus says "Make sure that the light you think you have is not really darkness." I hope this is for you and not me. It is my guess it is for both of us from time to time. We must pray for discernment. We might want to invoke Luke 10:42; it answers all. It says, "There is really only one thing worth being concerned about. Mary has discovered it." This was in response to Martha's complaints when Mary anointed Jesus' head with expensive perfume. If we will keep our eyes on Jesus and what He wants from us, all else will come together.

In Luke 8:10, there is reference back to Isaiah 6:9. Paraphrased it says: we read and do not understand and we hear but do not recognize the voice of the Spirit. I wonder, where will we be when He separates the wheat from the tares?

You may ask if I am saying sins are not to be judged. What would I say about murder? No, I am saying we need to look at the murderer. Did *we* play a part in his behavior? Was he getting back at life because he was taught that there was no hope for him? What happened along the way to lead him in this direction? Was it society? Who were the individuals in that society? Did he never want God because a well-meaning person, perhaps a Christian, made him think God could not possibly love him? How could God love any of us? It is only through His goodness and grace that the possibility exists. The murderer, because of his crime, must be punished. That must be. I will say, I have changed my mind about the death penalty, but I would put him away for life. I would not provide comforts, either! It is right that the murderer must pay, but what should be our part as society toward him? Should we forgive and desire that he comes to know God? Is that not the Christian way? What would Jesus do? What do we want to do with Paul? As I recall, Jesus spoke with him on the road to Damascus. He was on his way to commit additional murders of Christians. Think about it!

When was the last time we read Luke 7:27–36? This is the love your enemy stuff. We might need to read this every day. We seldom live by these words of Jesus. Sure, we love the lovable. It is the unlovable, however, whom this is talking about. Jesus follows this passage in Luke 7:37–42 with a discussion about condemnation. In verse 37, He says, "Stop judging others, and you will not be judged. Stop criticizing others, or it will all come back on you. If you forgive others, you will be forgiven." We do not like these words; we like our way a lot better.

We learn in the Bible that good trees produce good fruit, bad trees bad fruit. How many Christians, or churches, produce bad fruit? Do we run people away from salvation by the fruit of our members? I spent much of my life judging, although I said I wasn't. I was just letting others know what was right in accordance with the Bible. I find, however, that it was only those parts of the Bible I wanted to police! I pray I am not guilty of keeping someone from the kingdom. Again, the thought occurs that we as Christians are often seen as negative and judgmental, lacking love. We teach that God is love, but many of us do not live as if *we* love. It appears that love is left only to God!

Perhaps we need to read the gospels and truly study what they say to us. God is willing to provide wisdom when we ask Him to unfold what He wants us to understand. We need to get our priorities in order and take the time most of us are not willing to give. How much time do we spend *studying* His Word? Do we read the newspaper or watch television more often than we get out our Bibles? Luke 8:18 says, "So be sure to pay attention to what you hear. To those who are open to my teaching, more understanding will be given. But to those who are not listening, even what they think they have will be taken away from them." I like Luke and John. For more than thirty years, my favorite verse in the Bible has been John 8:36. I find it ironic because it means so much more to me now than before. In the King James Version, it says, "If the Son shall make you free, you shall be free indeed."

Are we free to make decisions about what denomination we are to join? My decisions about what denomination to join have changed through the years. Today, I am open to whatever ministers best to the individual. Whatever speaks truth and life is best. We must find those in whose presence we are transported to a level where we experience worship—worship for God—not worship for anything else. It must not be to choose a church where we make good contacts, or where we go just to have fun, or the church with the most clout, or the most money. Our choice for a church should be as important as our choice for a home. If it is not, we have missed something. We need to study to know what we believe; in so doing, we can choose our denominational preference. As I write that we need to do this, and we need to do that, I am reminded that much of this book is about judging and berating judgment. I am, and think I must, be judgmental to make each point! It is difficult to express one's viewpoint without a judgmental tone. I have to face the fact that all humanness or human nature, if you will, judges, even in preaching lack of judgment! We open our mouths, and judgment comes out. Yes, God has a lot of work left to complete in me, too!

There are various denominations, all believing they are the enlightened. All believe this is what the Lord has given them. You see,

I feel the same! Over the last year, I believe God has spoken to me about what He has been doing in my life—pretty narcissistic perhaps to say the Lord has set me apart. Has the almighty God chosen this person who tortured frogs (I do not believe I mentioned this anywhere else), this kid who did so many subversive things, a loner? God took this torturer, this loner, and set her apart for Him at about age fifteen. I believe that with all my heart. I did not know it, and it appears I have fought it most of my life. It is difficult to put all these thoughts and beliefs into words. Only if the words have come through inspiration will they make sense and be understood. I want you to recognize that although I had a meaningful, useful life, if my early years had dictated who I became, it is frightening who or what I might have become. I had trouble socializing, have committed more sins than I'm willing to tell the reader, and became an alcoholic, all in spite of God's intervention. Perhaps He allowed this, to show that anyone, just anyone, can be somebody. He will choose. What I do know at this moment is that I am laid far too bare with what I am saying to be comfortable. Silence, however, is not an option. It would be a lie! The right will reject me for being left, and the left will reject me for being right. Here I am, a misfit again! I did not want to put it on paper, but I was burdened to tell.

In going forward, I must say that I feel so certain, so very certain, that the Lord has spoken to me. No, He has not spoken in words, but in thoughts and dreams, from His Word, and through others. Therefore, I think I am right—yes, true enlightenment. I have THE WAY! There is only one problem; He has spoken to others whose enlightenment is different from mine! What do I do? Should I discount what I know to be truth, or should I discount their word? No, I remember a Scripture that reminds us God's ways are different from our ways. What are His ways? Obviously, it is to speak with us differently. You know what I notice? I notice that all enlightenment always points to Him! That is the key. He speaks to us at whatever level we can understand; i.e., to the level our ignorance can allow. If we need law, He gives us law as a basis. If we need love, He provides that as a basis. Whatever *we* need to find *Him*, He provides. Thus, we have the faiths we consider more fundamental, and those we consider more filled with love. He wants that none should perish. He tries to get us from every angle!

It is interesting to me how He took this law-based person and moved her to be a love-based person. I see more hope in love than in law. I see more of Jesus in love than in law. God loves us all whether we need law or love to see Him. Although I was and will continue to be a firm believer in strong discipline, I always disciplined in love. If discipline is to create change, it must be done in love! God, in my opinion, disciplines us in love; He alone should be the judge.

God knows our personalities. It appears to me that we need to accept all church denominations as those God has provided as a *way* to Him. He wants for none to perish. He knows us far better than we know ourselves. He may lay one thing on one person's heart and another on someone else's. One may need law to find the Son, another love. We must be open. We may not be right, but we need to realize that God is! It says to me that there are many church denominations all founded by well-meaning people. If each is sure of the word from God, it should indeed tell us something. It tells me that God leads us in different directions, but some try to place themselves in an equal position with God and judge others for their enlightenment. In so doing, I wonder how many unsaved we have run off from Christianity by our deep desire to make the rules for God. We fail to look at Jesus' example. Without realizing what we are doing, we often set ourselves up to behave like the Pharisees. As suggested earlier, we need to give *serious* thought to the fact that they were the ones who crucified Jesus. I'm grieved that we do the same.

In saying all this, do I believe my earlier, more rigid thinking was wrong? No, it was good for me at the time. Had I not had a foundation, whether law or grace, I think there would have been little hope for me to live a life anything close to the one I lived. Actually, there may have not been hope anyway except that God decided to use my life for His purpose. At this point I cannot truly say. I do believe I was supposed to be an educator, and perhaps some life was positively influenced because of me. I do not know whose it might have been, but perhaps it is truth.

At an earlier time in my life, I could not have understood my current thinking. That is certainly not to say that I now have higher thought. I believe it is simply in keeping with His current purpose for my life. I realize that in my past, I have been far too intent on what was right rather than recognizing that there may be fewer absolutes than I have thought. He wants *us*, not our religion!

Who then might be guilty of keeping us from seeking God's will for our lives, from loving Him and our neighbor? If we believe in the Bible, we believe in a deceiver, Satan if you will. He is said to be the prince of this world, and he must be very happy that many of us have made a mess of God's plan for our lives. Oh, how we have confused others, as well, in our confusion. Oh, how God must grieve!

Speaking of grieving God, what about doubt? From time to time, we all have doubts. We may not doubt the existence of the one true God, but something creeps in that makes us doubt something or another. At times, Christianity seems so preposterous, and we recognize why we must come as little children. As we age, it becomes so difficult; it seems so impossible for all this stuff to be true!

Like mine, every Christian life has probably experienced miracles, which proves that He's in the world, but we manage to explain them away. This time, I can't and I'm glad! This is a time in my life when, for the most part, people accept me. Some think I have gifts. It is a risk to bare my life on paper, but it is a risk I have to take because it may be what the Lord set me apart to do. What happens when all this is completed, I do not know. Only God has those answers. I know it is frightening to put it on paper, but I have to trust that He will take care of that as well. This message keeps coming to me. The reader has read it many times. Before you cast too many stones my way, please think about how you would feel if you were to bare your soul for all to see. This is the story of one that, at least until she was about thirty-five years old, perhaps even older, struggled to keep going. It is hard to admit that to myself, much less to place it on paper. It is frightening to think of all the negatives people might think now as they read. For the most part, my many weaknesses and general shortcomings have been hidden from others. After the book is in print, if that is what is intended to tell what He has done in my life, I do not know what if anything comes next. As stated earlier, I do not have a clue. I know I have been set apart for Him, and believe I have been during my entire life.

Chapter 18

LIFE WITH JESUS

A life without Jesus, I cannot imagine. As much as I have run from the many wonderful things that may have been a part of my life had I consciously sought to be in God's will, my path has always been with Him on the periphery. Partly because of my law orientation, I never felt that I was good enough to serve Him in a way that would really count for something. How could He use someone who smoked and could not quit? Later, I wondered how He could use someone who was an alcoholic and could not change. I did not know how He could use someone who was divorced and could not be sane in marriage. How could He use someone who was very shy and could not be friendly? How could God even want me, much less use me!

Had I not believed we had to be a certain way before God could use us, my guilt and fear may have been different. I never questioned that God loved me, I just could not understand why I was so weak. Why did I have all these problems in my life? Interestingly, most on the outside would have never known I had any problems!

Actually, I love people so deeply that it hurts! I want to reach out; I want to hug; I want to say I love you because I do. Even now with all my many years of growth, I continue to hold back when I want to go forth. My humanness gets in the way of His godliness!

What about you? Have you ever made a decision for Christ? Do you believe in Jesus? It all starts there. If you believe that Jesus is the Christ, the Son of the living God who came to earth, died on a cross for you, and rose on the third day, you have accepted Jesus as your Savior. Unfortunately, I think many calling themselves Christians stopped at this point. Believing in Christ may provide a ticket to heaven; I do not know. Previously, I would have said yes. Now, as most would think my beliefs have become watered down, I have begun to wonder if just saying you believe is enough.

My concern is not that believing is not enough. My concern is that we have convinced ourselves that because we attend church, or attended church at some time, or had some kind of spiritual experience some time or another that we are saved. Maybe so, but the Scripture in Matthew 7:14 states, "But the gateway to life is small, and the road is narrow, and only a few ever find it." This is certainly not a new Scripture for me, but I am looking at it differently. During this past six months, I have realized the real guidelines for living, and found that what we are usually taught is handpicked by those who want to play the we-know-it-all game. I certainly do not know it all: I only know what the Lord has unfolded for me. For most of my life, I have just accepted what I was told and read Scriptures with a preconceived knowledge of what they mean, in accordance with what I have been taught! How many of us do the same? You know, if we *really* want to know what they mean, we will study, asking (expecting to receive) for discernment from the Holy Spirit. The Bible says this works, but we have been brainwashed to believe it doesn't. Must we leave it to the scholars? No, scholars disagree. That is why we have a different denomination on every corner! This may be another area where we want to fit in so badly that we dare not think for ourselves (in accordance with the Spirit's leading). We think: who am I to *think* I have a hot line to the Spirit! Oh, what little faith we have!

In Acts 16:31 (KJV) Scripture says, "Believe on the Lord Jesus Christ and thou shalt be saved." That Scripture is cited on many occasions relative to what is necessary for salvation. This was Paul's answer when asked by his jailer while in prison what was necessary to be saved. In Luke 18:18–35, however, we read the story of the rich young ruler who asks Jesus what is required of him to be saved. Jesus tells him he needs not to murder, steal, lie, commit adultery, etc. The young man tells Him he has always observed the commandments, but Jesus tells him there is still one thing he lacks. He asks what that might be, and Jesus tells him to sell everything he has to give to the poor. The young man leaves very sad because he has so much wealth. A discourse follows that it is easier for a camel to pass through the eye of a needle than for people with wealth to go to heaven. It would appear that the greatest stumbling block we face is our lack of willingness to give wealth and possessions up here, to have them there. This brings me back to an earlier thought that we really do not truly believe that all this "Jesus stuff" is really the truth! What profession of Christ we do make is "just in case, as unlikely as it is, that it is truth!" If we really believed in eternity, we would give anything for it, yes, anything, including any amount of wealth we might have. What about someone we deeply love? Will we give them just about anything in our power if they want it? We will, and they cannot provide us with eternity! I think if we really believed, we would comb through the Bible with a fervency greater than anything else we have ever done, and prayer would be without ceasing. We might not need to give up wealth or anything else. We would only have to give up those things that separate us from Christ. For the rich young ruler, it was wealth.

All right, let's get back to being saved. It is the most important decision any person will ever make, that is, if the "Christian thing" is not a hoax. I promise; it is not a hoax! But, who am I? Jesus was the Son of God, and He was not believed! Oh, to be able to impart how *exhilarating* it is to walk with the Lord! There are times I almost feel I can touch Him. Of course, being human, there are times I wish He would draw near. I grieve when I feel He has gone away, but it always turns out that *I* have gone away.

Nothing, absolutely nothing, can equal the joy that communication with God brings. I know He loves me just like I am. I am a sinner saved by His grace. I am one who has fought just about everything terrible this world has to offer. I fought the world while praying and asking God to deliver me. He did deliver me when His time was right! I am a firm believer in God's timing. Anita, my wonderful roommate, used to talk about God's timing, and I could not understand. Unfortunately, it is like everything else we humans deal with: until we have something particular happen in our lives that helps us understand (and sometimes we do not even recognize it when it does happen to us), we often seem blinded to truth.

As I sit here typing at my computer, I am praying that God will inspire me, infuse me with something that will grab the unsaved reader to get a vision of something divine! Those words seem far out, but they are truth! Even as a teenager, I said the only reason we live on this earth is to determine where we will spend eternity. I have always believed that to be so, but it has become far more meaningful lately during my more intensive study of the Bible. We do not live as if our mission on earth is to determine where we will spend eternity! We live for comfort and pleasure! It might remind us of the rich young ruler. Such thoughts make me wonder what is truly required to be saved.

Keeping all the laws, which is impossible, cannot be the answer. One may say you strive to keep them. What a dreadful life! Why not strive to truly *serve* God and love your neighbor? If you truly treat your neighbor as you want to be treated, you will stay out of most trouble. We will fail whatever we try alone, because we will have a carnal body as long as we live on this earth, whether we like it or not, no matter *who* we are. We need the constant companionship of God to get us through. That is partly what is wrong with us now: we concentrate on the negative when we simply need to look to Jesus! The motto "What would Jesus do?" would be great if we would really live it. We do not seem to. We are too interested in the things of this world and being accepted by other people, and thus choose to continue moving down the path more traveled by, whether saved or not.

Thoughts, thoughts, and more thoughts come to my head as I seek to know what should be known about salvation. What if there really is an eternity that goes on forever? Fathom it for a minute. Where do you want to be? Forget, for the moment, everything the religions have told you about having to do, or being this or that. Ask Jesus to speak to you. He loves you. That is the truth. He loves you just as you are! He may not like some things about you. You don't like everything about yourself either! Tell Him you want to be open to what He wants to say to you. Tell Him you know you need His help. Tell Him you really want to love Him and be who He wants you to be. Tell Him you want to spend one day just loving Him and treating everyone you come in contact with that day like you want to be treated. Tell Him you feel so weak. Tell Him you want to be sure that He is real—you really need Him to make you know. At the end of a day after consciously living that entire day loving Him and treating others like you want to be treated, tell Him about the good things of the day and the failings of the day. Tell Him you want to try again tomorrow, but you can't try alone— you need Him. It can last forever if you choose!

As you move through each day, read the Bible. Ask for wisdom and understanding. By the way, as each day goes by, life may get harder and harder. The closer I get to God, the more problems I sometimes encounter. The only good thing? I have to lean that much more on Him to get me through. Remember each day, that life can be a struggle. I do not see it as a struggle to be good—I see it as a struggle to survive humanity! It seems that many humans are out to get us. Unfortunately, some are other Christians. Oh, that it were not so. They mean well. They are just trying to survive themselves! They are behaving the only way they know how. That is what religion often becomes. We need and long to be with other Christians and therefore have to just swim the tide the best we can, realizing the weakness of humanity. Bite the bullet, find a fellowship where you are comfortable. I say, be yourself. You may have to take more time in finding the congregation that is right for you, but when you do, it will be rewarding.

It saddens me so that religion has given Christianity such a bad name. Except for those folks who may have themselves fooled (I may have once been one of them through ignorance, and who knows, I may remain fooled), the thou-shalt-not types are far too much like the Pharisees and think Jesus loves them most. Jesus loves us all *equally*. We need to remember *that* above all else! The Pharisees had everyone stirred up in Jesus' day as well. We are known to Him by our fruit. The fruit I am seeing is that of helping our fellow man in need, loving the unlovable, and trusting Him to guide our lives, not berating others.

At the point you *really* believe Christ died for you, you are what some call born again. I tend to simply call it becoming a Christian. At any rate, when this takes place, you become part of the family of Christ through His Spirit. It takes on two aspects—one heavenly, one earthly. First Corinthians 12:13 says, "Some of us are Jews, some are Gentiles, some are slaves, and some are free. But we have all been baptized into Christ's body by one Spirit, and we have all received the same Spirit." In Ephesians 5:30, Paul says, "and we are his body." On earth, we embody His Spirit, whereas in heaven, we are His bride. What a deal! Your earthly family may get mad at you or even throw you out, but you remain part of your family whether you or they want it to be or not. It is the same with Christ's family: when His Spirit lives within you, no matter what you do, it remains! What a relief! Does that mean we want to sin because we can? No, we want to live close to our life, the Lord! That is when an understanding of *true* forgiveness and a life with Him begins.

I am so very glad I trust in Jesus rather than in mankind. Mankind would not give me a chance. It would be like the man in Matthew 18:21–35. It is the story Jesus gave Peter when he asked Him how often he should forgive someone who sinned against him. Jesus told him seventy times seven! The story He used to illustrate was about a king who was clearing his debtor books and called in a debtor who owed him millions. The debtor begged the king to be patient and he would pay it all back. The king decided to forgive the entire debt. After this man left the benevolent king, he went to one of his own servants who owed him only a few thousand dollars. He demanded payment immediately! His servant begged him to give him more time, but he was not willing and had the servant arrested and jailed. When the king found out what had happened, he sent for the unforgiving man and called him evil. He had forgiven him a very large debt, and although he was forgiven, he had been unwilling to forgive another of a far smaller debt. The king became angry and sent the first man to prison until he had paid all his debt. In verse 35 Jesus says, "That's what my heavenly Father will do to you if you refuse to forgive your brothers and sisters in your heart." I am indeed glad Jesus is our Savior and our fellow man is not. If nothing else is digested from this book, the one thing I would have all readers internalize is that Jesus took *all our guilt* to the cross, but man, so often a Christian, comes along and gives it back! Oh, how sad Jesus must be. Thank goodness, even the Christian who stumbles in this way, remains under grace and never experiences the guilt he lays on another.

Little positive about law has been said in this book. I do not see law as what the Lord has laid on my heart to talk about. I do, however, want it understood that I think morals are important, as well as justice and regard for authority. It greatly saddens me that our country has degraded itself without regard to its fellow man. It may partly be the result of a lack of love among Christians! Support for differences would probably not cure everything; but Christianity might take on a more desirable hue among the lost were we to support one another. We spend far too much time questioning others' beliefs when we could be spending that energy on leading people to God. Again I say, God wants *us*, not our religious affiliation. The deceiver wins again! I hope my reader does not believe that my discourse has been a slam against the more fundamental faiths. That is not true at all. Much of what I have as a basis of belief came from strict doctrine. I now belong to the Christian Church (Disciples of Christ) because it more nearly fits what I believe is right for me. However, I would not be who I am today without my earlier foundation coupled with my current church fellowship, so I praise God for a variety of choices. It matters not what our affiliations may be. For the third time I must say, God wants us and not our church denomination. My major concern is with Christians who want to judge, and we find that in every membership. Often, our judgment is for the small things! Judgment must be left to God. He told us to love and to leave judgment to Him. All of us come short of being worthy to cast stones. In our ranting about the degradation of the world, if all Christians had worked together, we might have wielded enough power to make things turn out differently. He knew we wouldn't!

It saddens me greatly that we have not banded together as Christians to stand for God in these difficult times. I could go on and on, but it is about time to come to the end of my ramblings. Before I come to a stop, I want to repeat the story of the Pharisee and tax collector as told by Jesus in Luke 18:10–14. "Two men went to the Temple to pray. One was a Pharisee, and the other was a dishonest tax collector. The proud Pharisee stood by himself and prayed this prayer: 'I thank you, God, that I am not a sinner like everyone else, especially like that tax collector over there! For I never cheat, I don't sin, I don't commit adultery, I fast twice a week, and I give you a tenth of my income.' But the tax collector stood at a distance and dared not even lift his eyes to heaven as he prayed. Instead, he beat his chest in sorrow, saying, 'O God, be merciful to me, for I am a sinner.' I tell you, this sinner, not the Pharisee, returned home justified before God. For the proud will be humbled, but the humble will be honored."

Pride has been a big stumbling block since the Fall. Satan has a good time with so much of our behavior. It is my opinion that Satan has a really good time with our taking shots at other Christian faiths as well. The Lord would want all denominations to support one another and not be divisive. Oh, how much power Christianity would wield in this world if we did not fight what may end up being minor differences! We let the deceiver win! We give little thought to the fact that Heaven will be made up of all denominations, but on earth we cannot seem to get along! What kind of support does that give our Lord?

It is my hope that your thoughts have been tweaked as you read this book. At times, it has been a labor of love. At other times, it has been a labor of fear. In about thirty minutes I will have spent fifty hours in front of the computer. The Lord, I trust it was He, filled me with words to put on paper. Every hour has been spent in prayer. I want more than anything to say *yes* to whatever God wants from me. I have begun to wonder if He doesn't sometimes just decide to "choose" someone to do something just because He wants to. After all, He is God and can do whatever He wants to do! I feel like that is what has happened with me. It certainly proves to me that there is nothing we can do to be good enough, or on the other hand, so bad that He doesn't want us. I know I think He had me write all this because He wants *you!*

While writing this manuscript I have come to love the imag-ined reader, and as much as I want to bring this to a close, I hate to say good-bye to you. So, say yes to Jesus, and look me up when we all go to be with Him!

To order additional copies of

Burdened ~~To~~ Tell

Have your credit card ready and call:

1-877-421-READ (7323)

or please visit our web site at
www.pleasantword.com

Also available at: www.amazon.com

Printed in the United States
33076LVS00005B/428